How to Feed Your Hyperactive Child

How to Feed Your Hyperactive Child

Laura J. and George E. Stevens
and
Rosemary B. Stoner

ILLUSTRATIONS BY
Anthony F. Holtgrefe

DOUBLEDAY & COMPANY, INC.
GARDEN CITY, NEW YORK

Acknowledgments

We wish to thank our mothers and mothers-in-law for their encouragement, enthusiasm, and recipes. Special thanks to Flo Stoner for her commitment to our idea for this book and for her tireless efforts trying out recipes. Thanks also to our many friends and neighbors who tested recipes, offered ideas and suggestions, and critically tasted many of the recipes in this book, and to members of our local group of Parents of Hyperactive Children for their personal experiences and encouragement.

Library of Congress Cataloging in Publication Data

Stevens, Laura J   1945–
How to feed your hyperactive child.

Includes index.
1. Hyperkinesia—Nutritional aspects.   2. Cookery
for hyperactive children. I. Stevens, George E.,
1936–   joint author. II. Stoner, Rosemary B.,
1941–   joint author. III. Title.
RJ506.H9S72   641.5′63

ISBN: 0-385-12465-1
Library of Congress Catalog Card Number 76–23799

*To Jack, Jeff, Diane, and Rob and all hyperactive
children, their siblings and parents*

Contents

Recipes for ingredients marked with an asterisk (*) may be located by consulting the Index.

Foreword

A pediatrician may receive many requests during the year for evaluation of a child with a "learning disorder," "minimal brain dysfunction," "RMBD," or "behavior problems." These children often have been tested and studied by the school system. Behavior modification approaches have been used with minimal amount of results. The parents often ask the physician's opinion because they are "at the end of their ropes." They come to the physician for immediate help to solve the behavior problems. The pediatrician does realize that comprehensive evaluation of each child is necessary if a long-term solution is to be found. This evaluation must include comprehensive medical history, psychometric testing, and a detailed neurological and medical evaluation. With answers from this above evaluation a good program may develop which will help alleviate the child's behavior problem.

Drug treatment has been found to be effective in many children with this behavior problem. However, some children do not respond to any known treatment. In 1973, Dr. Ben Feingold suggested that an additive-free and salicylate-free diet may be important to the treatment of these children. There have been scattered reports that indeed the diet has been helpful. The American Academy of Pediatrics in a recent publication has been unable to document this improvement, but a more recent study by a group of researchers at the University of Pittsburgh has cautiously concluded that an additive-free and salicylate-free diet may reduce hyperactivity in some children.

This volume has been published to assist parents in preparing meals for children who are on this diet treatment program. We would encourage any child who is placed on this diet to have a pediatrician or a physician follow him closely.

Wendell A. Riggs, M.D.

Introduction

No two hyperactive children are exactly the same. Their personalities, problems, strengths, and weaknesses are as varied as other children's. Generally they do tend to have several of the following characteristics: constant overactivity with no purposeful goal in mind, short attention spans, poor powers of concentration, unpredictable behavior, impulsiveness, inability to delay gratification of needs or demands, low frustration levels, explosive emotional outbursts, and poor performances in school.

So even though your hyperactive child is not exactly like our Jack, you will probably be able to identify with our experiences.

Jack arrived more than three weeks early after an easy delivery. He was a beautiful baby and we were thrilled with our first-born child. We hadn't been around kids much, but we were confident that parenthood would come easily to us both. When Jack's grandmother left for home after helping us out, she said wistfully, "Now do enjoy him!"

Enjoy him? Impossible. He cried more and more each day and finally raged with colic for nine long months. Nothing helped. We changed formulas, schedules, we burped him more frequently and we walked the floor by the hour. One visit the doctor said we were "obviously" not feeding him enough; the next visit he said Jack was "obviously" being overfed. The only "obvious" thing to us was his intense rage and pain—over what, we never knew. Nothing we did ever seemed to ease his distress, and as parents we felt worthless and rejected by this screaming, squirming little guy—not an unusual reaction to a colicky baby.

On the other hand, Jack did have many delightful times even during these colicky months. He was either very, very happy or very miserable and there weren't many moments in between. As he continued to develop, he had a ready smile, a happy laugh, and quite a sense of humor.

By the time Jack could sit up at six months he was in constant motion rocking back and forth. He continued this when he learned to stand and would rock by the hour. He also learned to bounce in his crib. Often he would awaken in the night and bounce for several hours and again when he wakened in the morning. Needless to say, he soon wore out one mattress, and then another. People downstairs complained that their ceiling went "thump, thump, thump" all the time. He even tried to bounce on the floor but found rocking back and forth easier.

He walked at eleven months and from then until after age three he would not cuddle or be held at all. He rejected all our efforts to be physically affectionate. While the doctor told us to stop his bottle at a year, we continued for several more months as those were the only moments we could hold him.

Although Jack babbled constantly when he was only a few months old, we waited and waited for his first words. He just continued to babble incessantly even alone in his crib. When he finally started to say some words, his speech was very hard to understand. We finally had him tested at a speech and hearing clinic when he was three and a half. Their diagnosis was normal speech development except his overactivity caused his words all to pour out at once making them unintelligible. This was one of our first clues that we had a hyperactive child.

Jack's early toddler years were perhaps his best stage, or maybe it was just that the colic had ended. He never seemed to go through the "terrible twos" but life had often been terrible with Jack. The older he got, the more he fussed and whined. Temper tantrums were frequent and intense. He raged over nothing. His behavior was completely unpredictable—happy one moment, sobbing the next, and often it was impossible to determine a cause. Potty training became a futile undertaking. Teaching him to dress himself was a wasted effort. Yet, he still had many delightful moments and basically had a happy disposition and was obviously very bright.

By the time he was three and a half, however, it was plain to us we had a child completely out of control. We had to do something. Thus began the many trips to specialists for help. He began nursery school, and although he wasn't a dropout, problems were increasing with his peers. We started to see a child psychologist. The psychologist told us Jack had a number of behavioral problems, but he was more concerned by Jack's extreme anxiety, tenseness, and overactivity. He urged us to use behavior modification to accomplish such tasks as potty training and dressing. Also he was a strong advocate of the "time out" room for temper tantrums, etc. We had little success with either technique no matter how hard we persevered. After six months we had made little progress. However, the psychologist's assurance that Jack's problems were not our fault was reassuring.

Shortly after Jack turned four, we took him to a pediatric neurologist at the nearest medical school. After examining Jack and taking a detailed case history, he confirmed that Jack was hyperactive in the medical sense of the word, that Jack's problems came from within him, and we were not the cause. Just hearing his reassurance again was comforting. He recommended we continue working with the child psychologist and placed Jack on Ritalin. He rarely used drugs, especially on preschoolers, but he felt Jack's case warranted such use.

Jack improved some on the Ritalin at first and life was more bearable for all of us. Within a few months, however, the effect wore off and the dose had to be doubled. This turned Jack into a Zombie—dull, listless, glassy-eyed. Although our hearts ached to watch his hyperactivity, we couldn't stand seeing him "drugged" either. The dose was reduced and again Jack improved. The improvement was short-lived. We were back to the "old Jack" plus undesirable effects of the medicine. Our new pediatrician, who has been quite supportive, tried another drug with no improvement. He and the pediatric neurologist concluded we would just have to learn to live with Jack's behavior as they didn't want to try other drugs.

We were desperate. Our family life was in a turmoil. We were worried not only about Jack but also about the effect on his brother who was almost two. We were mentally and physically exhausted. Learning to live with Jack's behavior seemed impossible—we'd been trying for four years.

In the midst of this despair, we read a book by Dr. Ben Feingold (see *Why Your Child Is Hyperactive,* Random House, 1974). Dr. Feingold argued that food additives can cause hyperactivity in some children. Our specialists took a dim view of this new concept, but we checked with our pediatrician and he agreed we had nothing to lose by trying the diet. In fact, he had other patients on the diet who had improved, some dramatically.

The diet theory made some sense to us from our previous experiences with Jack although we were unaware of their significance at the time. Jack's colic had begun when liquid vitamins (artificially flavored) were started. His colic subsided somewhat with the diet of formula, oatmeal, and bananas and worsened when the doctor insisted we reintroduce other foods. He had become markedly more hyperactive after taking artificially colored and flavored cough medicine and was obviously worse when we used artificially colored and flavored chocolate candies as rewards in potty training and in encouraging good behavior.

So we plunged full speed ahead into the diet. Within five days we could see an improvement. For the first time, we sat down with Jack and explained as best we could to a four-year-old what hyperactivity is, that it was not his fault or ours and that everyone wanted to help him to have happier days by not eating certain foods. Jack, who had never been reasonable in his life, accepted this calmly and had been amazingly good about the diet. The kids at nursery school accepted that Jack couldn't eat certain foods and no one made a fuss. The teachers were most co-operative.

After three weeks on the diet, we had a conference with his teachers. They were delighted and amazed by the changes in Jack. His attention span had increased, he had established eye contact when talking to other kids, and his interaction with the other children had improved tremendously. He no longer stormed over trivial matters. His speech had improved and could be more easily understood.

We were delighted to have the teachers confirm our observations. At home, Jack's days were much smoother. Gone were his terrible rages and tantrums. He could hold still to get dressed and started to put his shoes on by himself for the first time. He also could put his coat on with no help and would hang it up when asked. Previously, both tasks had always ended in Jack being so wild and frustrated that his coat would be thrown across the room and he would be screaming on the floor. Now he was obviously feeling good about himself and about us, as he was full of kisses and hugs for us all. He also could sit on our laps and cuddle without being thrown into a tizzy. We could reason with him for the first time ever.

This is not to say that Jack didn't have his ups and downs—all four-year-olds do. Furthermore, for over four years he'd learned certain ways to react to situations and this was unlikely to change overnight. However, the change has been dramatic and much more so than any he ever showed on drugs. Even when the drugs worked, there were still awful times before they took effect in the morning and after they wore off at night. Now we don't have those extremes. Instead, he's relaxed, calm, and happy.

We never doubted that the diet was responsible for the change. This was reinforced by several "goofs" we made along the way which are bound to occur from time to time. One night he had a restaurant hamburger with catsup, pickle, relish, and mustard. The next day the "old Jack" was back. By the following day, however, he had calmed down and started to improve again. One lesson we learned that day was that we would rarely knowingly cheat on his diet. The price was just too high. We have had other downs, but by carefully studying the diary of his food intake we have discovered the probable sources and removed them from future meals.

After six months on the diet we reintroduced one item we thought had really caused a reaction on the chance it had been just our imagination. It wasn't. Jack's hyperactivity returned. He was completely unable to reason. Much of his talk didn't make any sense. The "old Jack" had returned again. After forty-eight hours he calmed down and was fine. We hadn't seen behavior like that in months. In our mind, the only cause could be what we'd given him to eat. We happily returned to the diet knowing the extra effort and time were really worth it.

At first we had found the diet confusing, restrictive, and frustrating. When we saw the list of forbidden foods, we were overwhelmed. How could we eliminate all those foods from Jack's diet? We found our frustration was shared by other parents of hyperactive children (we had organized a local group of parents of hyperactive kids) who wanted to try the diet but were dumfounded when they saw the list of forbidden foods. They just didn't know where to start and how to stick with the diet long enough to see results. Thus was born the idea for this cookbook: to provide parents with "safe" recipes and menu suggestions to carry them through the most difficult early weeks until the diet became a way of life. We enlisted the aid of our sister-in-law, Rosemary Stoner, whose family was also on the diet.

Advantages of the Diet

The diet has many advantages over other forms of treatment. First, a doctor's close supervision may not be constantly required, except to ensure your child is receiving adequate nutrition. You and your child's teacher will be the best judges of whether the diet is really working or not. If your child is on medication, you will want to discuss with your doctor how to decrease the dosage if you are otherwise seeing improvements with the diet. Jack had been on a low dose of Ritalin, so we were able to withdraw it at the start of the diet. Many children, though, would need to have medication reduced gradually. For this, you will need your doctor's advice. He will probably be as delighted as you are to reduce the dosage or eliminate drugs altogether if you get successful results.

One wonderful advantage of the diet is that it is harmless *as long as you provide a balanced, nutritious diet.* Unlike medications, it should carry no possible long-term risks for your child, assuming you provide him with balanced meals. In fact, your child's diet (and your whole family's) should be more natural and more nourishing. If you have ever promised yourself to serve your family less junk and more nutritious meals, now is your chance. Food additives are not only being criticized these days for their effects on some hyperactive kids, but also some researchers feel many additives have not been sufficiently tested for safety. Some additives have been linked to cancers and birth defects in animals. Your diet should be more nutritious because you will have to take a very, very careful look at what your family is eating. Since almost all vitamin pills contain artificial colorings and flavorings, you will not be giving them to your child; instead, you will want to be sure he is getting all necessary nutrients from his foods. (See Appendix D for a short guide to basic nutrition.) In addition, you will be eliminating most of the "junk" foods from his diet as they are loaded with additives and offer little nutrition-wise.

Cost-wise you will probably find your grocery bill increasing at the start as you switch over to the "safe" foods. In the end, however, you will probably be saving money by buying fewer junk foods, more natural fruits and vegetables, and making some of your own staples.

Another advantage of the diet is that you will know quickly whether it's going to work or not. It is worth sticking to the diet for six weeks. By that time and probably much sooner (a week or so in some children) you will know whether it will work or not. Furthermore, the results should continue if the diet is faithfully followed. Many of the drugs work at the beginning and then their effects diminish. This should not be true of the diet.

The desperate parent who's tried everything or who dislikes the idea of medication has nothing to lose and everything to gain by trying the diet. No one can predict at this point which child will be helped. Not all hyperactive children improve on the diet. But it's worth a determined try for the sake of your child and the whole family.

Disadvantages of the Diet

There are some disadvantages to the diet. First, this diet has not been proven scientifically to the satisfaction of much of the medical community. Even Dr. Feingold says that he doesn't know why the diet works. But the mechanisms of many accepted cures and treatments in medicine are not understood. Only until more studies (several are under way and more are being funded) are completed will researchers be able to make the final judgment about the diet.

One major criticism of the diet from the scientific community is that it excludes some common foods which supply essential nutrients like many of the salicylate-containing fruits, good sources of vitamin C. You will want to be *sure* your child is receiving these nutrients *daily* in other foods. Check Appendix D or check the diet with your doctor or his nurse. You will also want to monitor your child's weight for any marked, continued changes. Report these to your doctor. However, if you serve a variety of foods to your family, there's no reason why your child should have any problem.

Another criticism of the diet is that any positive effects could be due to extra attention and time spent with the child preparing his meals and not to the diet itself. We have found that Jack rarely participates in preparing his diet and requires less attention now, but what time we do spend with him is more positive since he has calmed down. We look at it this way: who cares why the diet helps as long as the child gets better.

The diet is time consuming for the already harassed mother. Extra time is required for grocery shopping, menu planning, and meal preparation. Once you begin to think in terms of the diet and it becomes a way of life, the time factor diminishes. Furthermore, we found it took far less time to adhere to the diet rigidly than the previous amount of time required to steer Jack through the average day.

The diet is harder for the older child who spends most of his time at school and with his friends. He is used to all the "junk" foods and may be resistant to the whole idea. Without his cooperation, making the diet successful would be very difficult. If he can be guided through the first few weeks and can see the change in himself, he may become a very strong advocate of the diet. Most older children dislike having to take medication regularly or being teased about their school problems and all the other difficulties older hyperactive children have. They don't like their hyperactive behavior any more than their parents and teachers do. If the parent can choose a quiet moment to explain the diet and enlist his child's support and enthusiasm, there is much more hope for giving the diet a valid try.

Probably the hardest part of the diet is that it requires *strict adherence,* at least in the early weeks when parents are trying to discover if the diet is helping. If you can avoid it, don't knowingly disregard the diet. Even the slightest slip can set some kids off. As Dr. Feingold writes in his book:

> Compliance of 80 percent or 90 percent can lead to failure. It is important to remember that often a single bite or a single drink can cause an undesired response which may persist for seventy-two hours or more. An infraction on Sunday and then again on Wednesday may keep the child in a persistent state of disturbed behavior throughout the week.

If the diet has proven effective and the child has stabilized, then forbidden foods, one at a time, may be reintroduced over a period of time and the effects noted. At the start, however, don't cheat.

The Basic Diet (for the complete diet, see Appendix A)

There are several possible ways to approach this diet. First, you may want to start out by only excluding all artificial colorings and flavorings. If that alone doesn't change your child's behavior, then you will want to exclude all natural foods containing salicylates. Salicylates are aspirin-like compounds found naturally in some fruits and vegetables like apples, peaches, or tomatoes (see Appendix A for the complete list). If your child has ever reacted negatively to aspirin, then you will want to eliminate salicylates at the start of the diet.

Eliminate chocolate and cocoa at the beginning. We've talked with many parents of hyperactive children who are unfamiliar with the diet but already realize their children react to chocolate. It appears to be such a common problem (Jack reacted violently to homemade chocolate pudding) we recommend removing it at the very start. Carob will make an excellent substitute and chocolate can be tried again later on. We have included recipes containing chocolate for those children unbothered by it.

Also exclude any other food that "turns on" your child or to which you know he is allergic. These offenders may be completely natural foods. Instead of causing the usual allergic reactions of hives, runny nose, skin rashes, etc., these foods may cause a child to be hyperactive. Some of the most common problem foods seem to be milk, eggs, corn, wheat, sugar, chocolate (as mentioned above), potato, and members of the pea, bean, and soy family. But other natural foods could be the culprits too. How can you find these problems? First, your daily diary will help you pick out possible problems. Secondly, eliminate several of the most common problem foods for a week at a time. If your child improves, add the suspicious foods back, one at a time, until your child gets worse. Once you've found the problem, avoid that food for several weeks, then reintroduce it and see if your child can tolerate it once every few days.

If you still haven't noticed a change in your child or see only a slight improvement, then you may want to rid his diet of as many other additives as possible, like preservatives (BHA, BHT, etc.).

This sounds like a formidable task, but it really means just cooking with as many natural, fresh foods as possible. In particular, you may want to avoid bleached flour. Instead, use unbleached, naturally aged white flour or whole wheat flour.

Also, many pediatric medications contain artificial colorings and flavorings (aspirin, cough medicine, antibiotics, etc.). If medication is necessary, contact your physician and ask him to prescribe if possible only those which are uncolored and unflavored.

There are ways around some medication problems. Our pediatrician has been most helpful in selecting uncolored, unflavored drugs for Jack. Jack had a recurring ear infection and our doctor just prescribed a plain penicillin tablet. Later he prescribed another antibiotic that came in a colored capsule. We took the capsule apart and dumped the uncolored medicine in a little liquid. But do check with your doctor first, since not every drug should be removed from its capsule.

When we placed Jack on the diet, we eliminated foods in the order listed above. If we had to do it all over again, we think it would be faster and easier to take out salicylate foods and all possible additives at the very beginning. Once your child is stabilized reintroduce those foods containing additives or salicylates that mean the most to your child or are most convenient for you. These should be reintroduced one at a time every three or four days.

Evaluation of the Diet

When we started the diet, we soon discovered that we needed some method to evaluate Jack's day-to-day behavior as our days and weeks tended to blend together. We devised a grading system to evaluate his progress. Like all grading, this system is very subjective and influenced by factors other than the child's behavior. For us, however, the system was still helpful in noting progress or detecting "trouble foods." You may want to devise a system of your own or modify ours. See Appendix C for our grading system.

The Goals of Our Recipes

The recipes in this book stress (1) diet accuracy (2) appeal to children and teen-agers (3) easy preparation in a short amount of time (4) economy.

We wish we could guarantee instant, easy success for you and your child,* but, of course, that isn't possible. You may achieve dramatic results or you may have enough improvement to make life more tolerable. Or the diet may not help your child. But if you've tried everything else with little or no success and dislike using drugs, the diet is worth a try. Good luck!

* A special note on our use of "he," "him," and "his" when we discuss the hyperactive child. We have used these words for two reasons: first, because our experiences have been with a male child, and, second, because the great majority of hyperactive children are boys. We hope parents of hyperactive girls won't mind.

How to Feed Your
Hyperactive Child

1
Starting the Diet

Several factors are going to determine whether the diet will work for your child. First, you will hopefully be lucky and have a hyperactive child who is among the 50 per cent or so of hyperactive kids who respond to the diet. Second, your personal determination and dedication to trying the diet is vital. Third, your child's help will be crucial. And fourth, the attitude of the whole family will affect how you and your child view trying the diet.

At present there seems to be no way to predict which hyperactive children will respond to the diet. Dr. Feingold admits that it will not work for every child. There seems to be no correlation between children who benefit from medication and those who respond later to the diet. So, at least for now, there's no way of predicting beforehand whether your child will be helped. Keep your fingers crossed and plunge ahead!

That brings us to your role as chief cook and menu planner, whether you're the mother or father. If you're like most parents of hyperactive kids, you probably already feel harassed enough caring for your hyperactive child, other children, household chores, an outside job, or whatever. Now you've probably looked at the diet and are wondering how you can possibly cook for your family with all these restrictions. You can! Like any new diet, it will require a period of adjustment for both you and your family. The first few weeks are the hardest; after that, grocery shopping and cooking become much easier, your family has adjusted to slightly different meals, and hopefully your child is responding and his behavior is improving. Watching your child improve will lift your morale. As his hyperactivity and all its associated problems decrease, the physical and emotional strains on you will also decrease. So *hang in!* In our suggested menus (see Appendix E) we have purposely chosen for your first few weeks recipes that are easily prepared. You can adapt these to your family's likes and dislikes.

You'll want to choose a time that's good for both you and your child to begin the diet. A good start is so important for everyone's morale. Don't choose a hectic time when you are busy with extra activities, are planning a trip, or have guests coming. Instead, pick a relatively peaceful time for yourself. Some parents find vacation time from school a good time to start the diet as they feel they have more control over what their children eat. Other parents feel just the opposite way and find vacation time too hectic.

Now that you're determined to give this diet a try, you need to enlist the support of your child. Your approach will depend on his age and comprehension. Approach the subject in a positive manner. Expect him to be willing to co-operate and help. Jack, who had rarely had a reasonable day in his life prior to the diet, shocked us completely with his ability to understand what we were going to do. He had long been accustomed to drinking cola drinks as he wished, and we expected a terrible uproar when he learned he couldn't have them. Instead, he accepted this change matter-of-factly and has discovered many other drinks instead. So your child may very well surprise you with his attitude.

Choose a quiet, peaceful time to discuss the diet with your child, a time when his attention span will be long enough for you to tell him briefly what's going to happen. You will want to tell him some of the foods he will have to avoid, but you'll also want to stress those he can have that he particularly likes. He will eventually have to learn what foods he can't have but don't mention them all at the start unless he asks. Explain why he can't have them in terms he can understand. A young child can understand about artificial food colorings. Jack originally thought he couldn't have tomatoes because they were dyed.

You may want to explain your child's new diet in reference to other persons he may know who have to live on diets. This is an era of many different kinds of diets. Grandparents may be on low-fat diets or salt-free diets; parents may be trying to lose a few pounds; brothers or sisters may be allergic to certain foods; a relative or friend may be diabetic. Explain that his diet will help him to have happy, calm days.

If co-operation from your child is going to be difficult, you may want to set up some sort of reward system. These rewards might be inexpensive toys or maybe a trip to the park or zoo that you've been putting off, or some other special occasion with just you and your child. You know your child better than anyone, so you'll know best what will appeal to him. Older children in particular have so many opportunities to have snacks away from home that you can't possibly police them. Instead, tell them you expect them to turn down these treats for the time being. However, ask your child to tell you if he has had something forbidden so that you'll know. Promise not to be angry and then react as you promised if that occurs. Thank him for telling you, let him know that you appreciate his help and co-operation, that you know the diet isn't easy. But don't scold him or you'll discourage him from telling you another time.

You should also stress to your child that some of the forbidden items may be only temporarily withdrawn from his diet. Once your child has improved and has stabilized, you'll be able to reintroduce one item at a time and note any adverse reaction.

You'll also need to enlist the help of your spouse and any other children at home. In most families, the diet will only work if the whole family sticks to it. However, there's no reason why your other children can't buy their lunch at school and eat what they can't have at home. The same goes for the husband and/or wife at work. When you and your spouse go out together, you can order Italian food for a special treat or choose whatever you miss the most. At home, your family will be delighted with the substitutions you can easily provide for forbidden items. Simple gelatin desserts are delicious. Cranberry gelatin looks and tastes just like the store-bought cherry gelatin. But it's uncolored, more nutritious, and just as easily prepared. Same goes for popsicles, puddings, etc. No one need suffer on this diet.

You'll want to make it clear to other kids in the family that you won't tolerate any teasing connected with the diet. Once you've gotten into the diet, it's probably best not to discuss it very much. Treat the subject matter-of-factly. Just put the food on the table and don't discuss anything that's missing. The bigger the deal that's made, the harder the diet becomes for everyone. As your hyperactive child calms down, every family member will be much happier and more relaxed.

While you've been preparing yourself, your child, and the rest of the family for the diet psychologically, you'll also need to start becoming a "label reader." Start with your own cupboards and the foods your family eats most often. Are they artificially colored? Are they artificially flavored? Which foods contain salicylates? Do they contain preservatives? Some families feel it's worth the extra cost just to discard the foods they already have containing these chemicals. Or maybe a neighbor could use them or might be willing to pay you for some of them. Otherwise, use them up before starting the diet. When they need to be replaced (if they do), replace them with "safe" brands or substitutes—uncolored butter for margarine, grapefruit, pineapple, lemonade, etc., for orange juice. If you've been buying a lot of junk food, *stop!* In other words, get *all* of the foods not permitted out of your cupboards and refrigerator. You will need to read labels as you shop—we'll get to that in a minute.

Now is a good time to start keeping a detailed daily record of all food and beverage intake, including amounts eaten, brands used, etc. Keep a notebook in the kitchen and get in the habit of writing down after each meal or snack what your child has eaten. If your child has eaten away from home, be sure to ask what he's had. If he's old enough and can co-operate, get him to write it down. You'll also want to write down comments on his behavior. Otherwise, you'll forget just how he did behave on a given day. If you're going to start some evaluation scheme (see Appendix C), start now so you get a feel for it. Under our system, prior to starting the diet, Jack's "grades" would have fallen in the low C and D range most days. For us, these "grades" were helpful in giving us some idea of past behavior. Of course, this grading is very subjective and your own daily attitudes will color the results. But you do need some way to record how one day or week differed from another, as they all tend to blend together when you're tired and busy. You're going to be searching for clues like a detective, trying to discover what sets your child off. Since a natural food could bother your child too, your detailed diary and evaluations will help you find the culprit.

As you look for "safe" brands to replace those you've been using, you may find the list of products (see Appendix B) we've compiled helpful. Although companies may change their ingredients, those whose products are listed have assured us they are "safe." If you can't find these brands locally, you may have to write or call some other companies in your area asking for information. We've found almost all companies most co-operative and helpful even though their products were some we couldn't use.

You may also want to start planning your menus now. We were never "menu planners" on paper, but such a system could keep you from running into dinnertime without any ideas. We've included suggested menus in Appendix E. They are geared to providing balanced meals easily prepared with leftovers for lunches and other dinners. Good planning will save you much time and effort. Once you've discovered a recipe your family likes, make it in quantity.

This diet is very nutritious as long as you provide a variety of foods (see Appendix D). Don't fall into the trap of feeling so sorry for your child that you do nothing but stuff him with snacks, desserts, and candy. He needs balanced meals.

You'll also want to start making any staples you'll need (see Chapter 2) but can't safely buy. If you have a large freezer, you can freeze other things you'll be needing.

Now let's go grocery shopping for a minute. Actually, when you do go, plan to spend some time reading labels and getting ideas. Later on, this will go quite quickly as there will be many items you'll automatically pass by. Shop without your kids if possible. Otherwise, it will take twice as long and your concentration will be interrupted. Later on, your hyperactive child may learn to be quite helpful with the shopping and read labels as carefully as you. Sound impossible? Wait and see!

Okay, let's start shopping. We're going to go row by row as our own supermarket is laid out. First, we come to the packaged, processed luncheon meats. Artificial colorings and flavorings prevail. So do preservatives. There will probably be nothing that you can purchase from that array. We have seen in a health food store one brand (see Appendix B) of frozen additive-free hot dogs and bologna, which contain no preservatives. Maybe you'll be able to locate some; hot dogs are dear to most kids' hearts and there's no practical way to duplicate them at home. You'll want to bypass canned hams too. On to the frozen fish and poultry. Don't buy the self-basting turkeys. Read the labels on the fish. Try to find brands with nothing artificial added. Watch the breaded coatings on the prepared fish. You have no way of knowing if the flour is bleached or not unless you check with the manufacturer.

Over to the fresh meat department. The fresh meat and poultry are all fine. Choose what you want. However, note the purple stamping (concentrated grape juice) on the outside of some of the meat cuts. Jack seems to react to it, and the stamping is ground right into the ground beef. Explain this problem to your butcher and ask him to grind your meat without any stamping. We generally wait for a sale on round or chuck. Then we phone the store in the morning, tell them how much we need, and they grind it at the end of the day after they've washed the machine so it is free of all stamping. You will pay nothing extra for this service and your meat will taste fresher too. On your other meat cuts, trim away all the stamping before you cook them even if you have to remove a little meat with the fat. Unroll your rolled roasts to check if the stamped fat has been rolled up inside. Roll them back up and tie with string.

Unless you know someone in your store's deli section, it's best to pass up their food. You just can't tell what may be in it. Our next aisle has candy on one side, pasta products on the other. Forget the candy and gum. Even marshmallows are artificially colored! We've listed several candies we've found to be okay. Otherwise, you'll want to make your own if your child is really a candy fan. It's fun and he'll want to help. A candy thermometer will be a handy investment. Pasta products like noodles and spaghetti are generally made from wheat that is not treated in the same way pastry flour is. Pasta products, however, are not required by law to list their ingredients. They must list artificial colors and flavors though. As far as what to put on the noodles and spaghetti, that's another problem. Forget all the tomato-based sauces for now—tomatoes contain salicylates. Macaroni and cheese you'll want to make at home. Don't buy the prepared packages. We've included several delicious substitutes for tomato sauces on pasta, so don't despair. Rice is fine but beware of any prepared mixes.

Next come the canned meats, fish, and soups. Many brands of tuna fish and salmon are okay. Forget the hash, meat spreads, stew, etc. You'll want to make your own soups if they're important to your family. Most prepared soups are taboo on several accounts—tomatoes, artificial colorings, flavorings, etc. You'll find homemade soups delicious and easily prepared. On the other side of the aisle are the crackers and cookies. We've listed a few safe brands. Again, many are artificially colored and flavored and use bleached flour.

As we go down the next aisle, there are beverages like coffee, tea, and cocoa. Tea contains salicylates. Coffee should be okay if your child likes it. Some parents feel coffee calms their hyperactive child. Avoid the cocoa and chocolate drinks. If they have a carob drink, that should be okay. On the other side of the aisle are the condiments. Catsup is out, but we're providing several good substitutes. Cucumber pickles are out; other pickles that might otherwise be okay are often colored bright colors. Read the labels. Check the next chapter for making your own pickles. Several brands of mustard, mayonnaise, and salad dressing are okay. Or make your own. They're easily prepared and much cheaper.

Now we come to canned fruits and vegetables. You'll want to check the labels but most canned vegetables are fine if they don't contain tomatoes in any form. Some beans are colored. Non-salicylate fruits are fine too. But many of the drinks (bottled or dried) are a disaster. They're either artificially colored or flavored or both. There are some safe canned or bottled brands you'll want to locate—additive-free grapefruit juice, pineapple juice, pear nectar, and cranberry juice cocktail. These are good sources of needed vitamin C.

Cereals are a real problem for many kids. Most of the popular ones have coloring, flavorings, and preservatives. There are a few brands that are okay and manufacturers seem to be offering several lines of "natural cereals." Read the labels and choose carefully. Some groceries are beginning to stock additive-free corn flakes. Instant breakfast drinks are out.

You'll want to bypass the cake mixes, prepared icings, piecrust mixes, biscuit mixes, gelatin mixes, puddings, etc. Even angel food cake mixes have artificial flavorings and piecrust mixes are artificially colored. Unflavored gelatin is fine and a boon in cooking many things. You'll probably want to locate a 100 per cent pure maple syrup. It may be expensive, but you can always mix it with other kinds of syrups to stretch it as suggested in the next chapter. You should encounter no problems in buying sugars—confectioners', granulated, brown. In the flour line, buy unbleached white or the more nutritious whole wheat, soy, rye, etc.

Read the labels on any spices you buy. Most will be fine. Avoid cloves, as stated in the diet. Also allspice, as it's often made partially from cloves. Buy only *pure* extracts—vanilla, lemon, and lime if you can find it. Almond extract is out. Obviously no food colorings—you can make your own if needed by following the easy directions in the next chapter. Read the labels on any coconut you wish to buy and choose brands without additives. If you're going to buy any chocolate, buy the additive-free unsweetened brands or Baker's German Chocolate. These are pure. However, it's best to eliminate chocolate at the start of the diet as it seems to be a very common problem. If your store carries carob powder, it will make an excellent substitute for any recipe using chocolate. Don't buy the chocolate chips or other kinds of chips either. Buy nuts without preservatives.

Next come the soft drinks. Buy only the ones listed in Appendix B, unless you're sure they are naturally flavored and uncolored. Even the brands we've listed do contain other additives—but no artificial colorings or flavorings. The powdered drink mixes have both artificial colorings and flavorings.

Help yourself liberally to the non-salicylate fresh fruits and vegetables. But no tomatoes or cucumbers. No apples, peaches, oranges, grapes, strawberries (see Appendix A for the complete list). A few words of caution. First about the vegetables. Occasionally sweet potatoes are dyed. When vegetables like zucchini and green peppers appear to be waxed, either peel or scrape them well. The more you control precisely what goes into your child, the greater your chances of discovering what turns him on. In the fruit line, citrus fruits are often waxed—especially lemons and limes. They are fine for juice and inside pulp, but don't use the peels or rinds for anything unless you're positive there's nothing added. Occasionally some citrus fruits are injected with preservatives, but that information has to be stated on the packing cartons.

Many parents find these salicylate-containing foods the hardest to give up. They also contain valuable vitamin C. Don't despair. Once your child has stabilized and is doing well you can reintroduce them one at a time. Many hyperactive children don't seem to be bothered by them. We are also suggesting substitutes to be used in the meantime. You don't have to give up your pizza or your spaghetti just because you can't use tomatoes. Butter and cheese make a delicious spaghetti sauce. Pesto sauce made from sweet basil also makes a delicious substitute. At our house, we serve both pesto and tomato pizzas, but Jack is quite happy to stay away from the tomato. This may or may not work at your house. Jack also likes the rhubarb catsup so again we just serve both.

We also discovered that pears taste much like apples and can replace them in pie, applesauce, applesauce cake, etc. Likewise, cranberries taste like tart cherries besides looking the same. Some families have found they can serve orange juice as always but give the hyperactive child something else. We've all discovered fresh fruits we rarely used before—like papayas. Jack thinks it's great fun to buy a fresh pineapple. By the time it's cut up, everyone's devoured it. So give your family a chance to adjust to the new diet.

On to the dairy case. White milk is fine. Don't use chocolate. Buttermilk is fine but don't buy the kind with butterflakes added because the flakes may be colored. Margarine and butter are both colored usually with natural vegetable dyes but you will want to find an uncolored butter. Manufacturers add coloring to butter to standardize the yellow shade, as the color of the butter varies with the time of year and whether the cows are grazing in the pastures or eating in the barn. We have included in Appendix B one national brand of butter that is uncolored. Dairies are not required by law to list whether butter contains coloring or not. Likewise, with cheeses and ice cream. They too may be dyed or bleached and not state such information on the package. Blue cheese sometimes derives its color from dyes. So consult Appendix B or talk to your local dairy. It's possible you may be able to ask the dairy to sell you some butter or cheese before the dyes go in. Also check with any local specialty cheese stores. They often have a larger selection of uncolored cheeses and are more willing to find out their ingredients for you. Their prices may be higher however. In buying sour cream, whipping cream, cottage cheese, and yogurt, choose brands with the fewest additives. You'll also find yeast cakes in the refrigerator case. They don't contain preservatives like some brands of dry active yeast. Avoid all the ready-to-bake roll and cookie doughs. Also avoid any prepared gelatin molds, potato salad, cole slaw, and similar foods.

In the non-food aisle of cleaning products, we have two suggestions to offer. If your child is at an age where he still likes to drink water out of the bath and you use colored, scented soaps, you may want to switch to a plain, colorless, glycerine-type soap bar. This works well for shampoo too. You may want to consider avoiding aerosols around your child at the start. Jack accidentally got hold of some aerosol foot powder, pretended it was hair spray, and seemed to turn on until his hair had been thoroughly washed.

In the bread department there seem to be a few safe possibilities as listed in Appendix B. Some breads are dyed to look darker. Yellow dye is added to many baked goods to give the illusion of a product rich in eggs. You may wish to check with your local baker and find out if his white flour is unbleached. There are several frozen breads available that appear to be okay. Or you may wish to make your own breads as we've been doing so that you know exactly what ingredients are used. Maybe you're already good at this. If not, it's easy to learn and the great tasting, nutritious bread is worth the extra time. We're providing some super-easy, fail-safe bread recipes in Chapter 3.

One problem with the jams and jellies is that they may contain no artificial colorings, flavorings, or preservatives but do contain pectin for gelling purposes. Pectin is often derived from apples, so these jams and jellies should be avoided. Don't add pectin to your own jams and jellies. In the next chapter we're including jam recipes that will thicken without pectin and are easily prepared. Choose natural honey freely and in the peanut butter line choose brands with the fewest added ingredients—additive-free brands are becoming more available.

In the freezer case, choose unbuttered vegetables and non-salicylate fruits. Frozen vegetables have a higher vitamin content than canned vegetables. In the ice cream line there are a few natural brands available. Ice cream cones contain artificial colors and flavors, but it's fun and easy to make your own. Forget the popsicles—they're colored and flavored artificially. But you can easily and inexpensively prepare your own as described in Chapter 12. Ice cream is also easily made at home and is a fun project for the whole family. Don't expect it to last very long—it tastes too good. Also avoid frozen or other prepared whipped toppings. You can easily whip your own and for less money too. Frozen non-salicylate fruit juices are good but be sure to check the labels. Frozen lime juice is often colored.

You'll soon find that your grocery shopping goes quickly. So many areas you'll just pass by and in the other areas you'll know what brands are safe.

What about cost? Grocery bills seem to go up at the start of the diet as you replace many staple items. In the long run, however, your bills should decrease as you make more things from scratch, use few prepared convenience items, and avoid the costly junk-type foods. As you learn what your family likes, you'll be able to buy fruits and vegetables in season and items on sale. If you've done much home canning or freezing or have a large freezer, you'll find these talents and equipment helpful. However, you can also manage quite well without them. We had never done any canning before, do not have a freezer, and have managed just fine.

If you want even more information to help you in your shopping, you may wish to peruse *The Supermarket Handbook* by Nikki and David Goldbeck (Harper & Row, 1973). It's interesting reading and gives considerable information on various brands of just about everything.

Sticking with the Diet

Once your child has calmed down and you and your family are getting used to the diet, you need to stick to it. Here are some pointers based on our experiences with Jack and those of other families we know.

If your child is older, he may realize himself how much better he feels. If he's been on medication and your doctor has been able to reduce the dosage or eliminate it altogether, your child will no doubt be delighted with that. That will be incentive to continue the diet. But expect some times of rebellion. These children especially seem to want to eat everything forbidden when they've gotten off the diet at some point and are turned on again. They seem to lose their ability to reason. This has happened several times to Jack. When your child comes in angry and announces that he's tired of the diet and is going to eat everything in sight, don't lose your cool. Instead, use some psychology. Don't react by saying "Don't you dare do that again or I'll . . ." whatever you might feel like threatening. Instead, say something like, "You must be very tired of the diet. I know you miss many of the foods. I wish you could have them too." This type of response shows your child you understand how he feels and will likely calm him down. Don't make him feel guilty either by telling him all the extra trouble you're taking—he'll realize you're trying to help him.

There will be times when he'll either deliberately or unknowingly have things he shouldn't. Don't get angry and make a lot of threats. Just hang in until his behavior calms down again. There may be occasions when you feel it's worth the price you may all have to pay to let him go ahead and eat what he wants on a special day—a birthday, Easter, Halloween, or whatever. However, we will give you lots of holiday suggestions (see Chapter 14) so that you can plan special days for him without a lot of work and still stick to the diet. After-school snacks at friends' houses may be a problem. Try to encourage your child to bring his friends home for snacks and then provide them with lots of "safe" foods. Don't comment about the diet. See Chapter 12 for snack ideas that don't take much work. Be sure to include some treats in his diet—favorite desserts, some homemade candy, or whatever might encourage him.

Once your child has stabilized you'll want to reintroduce into his diet both those foods he misses most and those that make your cooking and meal planning easier. Start with the salicylates. Many hyperactive children don't seem bothered by them. If you've been excluding other additives like preservatives, try them again. Be sure to try only one new food at a time. But when you reintroduce this food, you might as well serve it in a large quantity or several times in a day or two so that you'll really know whether it causes a problem or not. If it does cause a problem, it may be that your child can tolerate just a little of it occasionally but not a steady dose.

You will want to continue to ensure that your child is receiving adequate nutrition from his meals. Is he eating a variety of foods? Is he getting all the protein, vitamins, and minerals needed? Is he getting vitamin C daily? Check Appendix D on nutrition. Continue to check his weight. If you are unsure whether he is getting adequate nutrition in his diet, or if his weight changes very much either way, consult your physician. Although Jack's appetite decreased, he gained several pounds the first few months, then leveled off at a healthy gaining rate. Don't be surprised if your child skips some meals altogether during the early weeks. Jack had never missed a meal prior to the diet, then, as his activity level decreased with the diet, so did his appetite (which had always been enormous). Again, if your child continues to skip meals or lose weight, consult your doctor. Otherwise, don't show concern or try to force him to eat.

What about eating out? This can be a problem when you visit grandparents or other relatives who may not understand. If possible, depending on your family situation, you should try to have them serve what your child can eat. Some grandparents don't like to acknowledge that their grandchild is hyperactive since it's something new to them and not understood. Too, they may like to serve lots of goodies. They think it's part of grandparenting. You will just have to be firm and emphasize how important the diet is for their grandchild. If they've seen much of him and can now see a change in his behavior, they'll be more inclined to go along with the diet. Do try to avoid a fuss about it or much discussion of the diet with your child present as it may just make things harder for him.

Eating in restaurants is another problem since you can't possibly see what goes on in the kitchen. Try to order plain items—a plain hamburger (bring your own bun if possible), a chopped steak, roast beef, roast turkey or chicken, lamb chops, pork chops, baked potato, cottage cheese, etc. It's harder at a hamburger stand —a plain hamburger is about the best you can do, with french fries, a clear soft drink or plain milk.

If your child has been receiving professional counseling, certainly don't stop until you're sure your child is coping well and overcoming his previous problems. Ask your doctor's or counselor's advice. Your child may need some time to mature, catch up in school and at play with his peers, and adjust at home. This can be harder for the older child whose problems have gone on longer. On the other hand, your child may surprise you with his new ability to cope better and be relatively unscarred by his hyperactive years.

If your child does not respond to the diet at all, at least you gave it a good try. Much research continues into hyperactivity, its causes and controls. One day there will be an answer for your child too; soon, we hope.

2

Making Your Own Staples

Recipes for making your own staples are included here to help you in several ways. First, you will need certain recipes until you have located "safe" products in your own area, such as uncolored butter, safe mustard, mayonnaise, etc. Until you're positive that you've found these items additive-free or have been assured by the manufacturers that they are "safe," these recipes will help you start the diet. Once you've located uncolored butter, you won't want to continue making it. It's expensive and time-consuming. Other products like mayonnaise and mustard are easily prepared at home and more economical too, although you may decide to save time by buying "safe" brands. (See Appendix B for some safe brands.)

Secondly, many of these recipes are intended to provide substitutes for forbidden items. Since tomatoes are taboo, and catsup is dearly missed by many kids, we've included several alternative recipes. Many hyperactive children seem to "turn on" on chocolate, so we've provided many recipes using carob bean powder as a substitute. While the taste of carob is not identical to that of chocolate, it certainly makes a good substitute for the chocolate fan and should not cause the same adverse reaction. It may also be used safely by those children allergic to chocolate.

Thirdly, we recommend using some of these recipes all the time for items whose ingredients may vary or are impossible to determine, like bread crumbs and croutons. It's also difficult to find additive-free broths, so basic recipes for those are included. Since all commercial food colorings are strictly forbidden, recipes for making your own natural colorings are provided.

Finally, other basic recipes are provided for your convenience so you'll have all you need at your finger tips.

Homemade Butters

HOMEMADE SALTED BUTTER

Makes 8 ounces

1½ pints pure whipping cream, chilled
1 teaspoon salt

Using an electric mixer on high speed, beat the chilled cream until it passes the foamy stage and begins to look like corn meal mush. Continue beating until lumps are corn-kernel size.

Drain off the liquid (this is buttermilk). Run very cold water over the remaining butter and press with a wooden spoon squeezing out more buttermilk. Discard the liquid and repeat procedure until the buttermilk is completely gone.

Add salt and mix thoroughly. Pack into containers and store in the refrigerator. Butter may be frozen up to six months.

STRETCHED BUTTER

Makes 16 ounces

2 teaspoons unflavored
   gelatin
2 tablespoons cold water
½ teaspoon salt
1 cup whole milk or
   evaporated milk

8 ounces Homemade
   Salted Butter* or
   uncolored store butter,
   softened

Soften gelatin in cold water. Dissolve thoroughly over hot water. Add dissolved gelatin and salt to milk. Gradually whip milk into the softened butter with an electric mixer until milk is entirely absorbed.

Pack into containers and refrigerate. May also be frozen for up to 6 months.

WHIPPED BUTTER

Makes 1½ cups

2 sticks uncolored butter, softened
¼ cup pure whipping cream
1 teaspoon salt

Beat softened butter with mixer on high speed until smooth. Slowly add the cream and continue to beat until well mixed and very light. Add salt and mix well. This stretches the butter and also makes it easier to spread.

HONEY BUTTER

Makes 1 cup

½ cup uncolored butter, softened
½ cup pure honey
½ teaspoon salt (if using unsalted butter)

¼ teaspoon cinnamon (optional)
¼ teaspoon nutmeg (optional)

When butter is soft, beat in honey and spices and whip until fluffy. Refrigerate and use as a spread on toast or biscuits, or melt and pour over hot pancakes, waffles, or French toast.

Basic White Sauces

THIN WHITE SAUCE

Makes 1 cup

For vegetables, soup, or macaroni.

1 tablespoon pure vegetable oil or uncolored butter
1 tablespoon unbleached flour

½ teaspoon salt
1 cup milk
Dash of pepper

(See cooking directions under Thick White Sauce* below.)

MEDIUM WHITE SAUCE

Makes 1 cup

For meats, eggs, noodles, fish, scalloped dishes.

2 tablespoons pure
   vegetable oil or
   uncolored butter
2 tablespoons unbleached
   flour

½ teaspoon salt
1 cup milk
Dash of pepper

(See cooking directions under Thick White Sauce* below.)

THICK WHITE SAUCE

Makes 1 cup

For soufflés or thick cheese sauces.

3 tablespoons pure
   vegetable oil or
   uncolored butter
4 tablespoons unbleached
   flour

¼ teaspoon salt
1 cup milk
Dash of pepper

Blend oil (or melted butter) with flour and seasonings in a heavy saucepan. Add milk gradually. Cook quickly, stirring constantly, until mixture thickens and bubbles.

Condiments

CATSUP I (TOMATO-LESS)

Makes 2 cups

1 quart (4 cups) fresh or
  frozen (thawed)
  chopped rhubarb
½ cup water
¼ cup chopped onion or 1
  tablespoon dried minced
  onion
1¾ cups packed brown
  sugar

¼ cup white distilled
  vinegar
½ teaspoon salt
¾ teaspoon ground
  cinnamon
½ teaspoon ground ginger
¼ teaspoon nutmeg

Combine rhubarb, water, onion, sugar, and vinegar in a heavy
2-quart saucepan. Boil slowly until thick, stirring frequently. Add
salt and spices, cook 5 more minutes. Cool. Put in blender to remove lumps and until consistency is equivalent to that of tomato
catsup.

Refrigerate in covered container. Use as needed, or pour boiling
hot into sterilized canning jars, leaving ⅛ inch space at the top.
Adjust lids. Process in boiling water bath for 5 minutes.

CATSUP II (TOMATO-LESS)

Makes 2 cups

2 cups fresh or frozen
  (thawed) cranberries
1¼ cups water
2 tablespoons dried minced
  onion
1 cup granulated sugar
½ cup brown sugar
¾ cup white distilled
  vinegar

2 teaspoons salt
1 teaspoon ground
  cinnamon
1 teaspoon nutmeg
½ teaspoon ground black
  pepper

In a large saucepan, cook berries in water until boiling. Reduce heat and simmer slowly until berries burst and become soft. Pour into blender and purée. Return mixture to saucepan and stir in remaining ingredients. Bring to a boil. Reduce heat but continue boiling, uncovered, for about 30 minutes, or until mixture thickens. Sauce will thicken more when cooled. Remove from heat. Refrigerate in a covered container or pour boiling hot into sterilized canning jars leaving ⅛ inch headspace. Adjust lids. Process in boiling water bath for 5 minutes

HORSERADISH

Horseradish roots
White distilled vinegar

Wash, scrape, and grate fresh horseradish roots. Fill sterilized canning jars two thirds full with grated roots. Fill jars to top with vinegar. Seal. Store in cool, dry place.

HORSERADISH SAUCE I

Makes 8 ounces

1 cup dairy sour cream	½ teaspoon dry mustard
2 tablespoons	¼ teaspoon salt
Horseradish,* drained	Dash of paprika

Combine all ingredients and mix well. Chill.

HORSERADISH SAUCE II

Makes 8 ounces

8 ounces softened cream cheese
3 tablespoons Horseradish,* drained
1 tablespoon pure lemon juice

Whip cheese. Add horseradish and lemon juice. Mix well and chill.

MAYONNAISE

Makes 16 to 18 ounces

2 egg yolks
3 tablespoons white
   distilled vinegar
1 teaspoon sugar
1 teaspoon salt

Dash of pepper
1 teaspoon dry mustard
½ teaspoon paprika
2 cups pure vegetable oil

Place egg yolks with 1 tablespoon vinegar in mixing bowl and whip with an electric mixer. Continue beating and add sugar, salt, pepper, mustard, and paprika. Add oil a tablespoon at a time, beating continuously until mixture is very thick. Beat in remaining vinegar. Gradually add remaining oil and beat until mayonnaise is thick and well blended. Refrigerate.

HOT MUSTARD

Makes 2 cups

1 cup white distilled
   vinegar
1 cup dry mustard

2 eggs
1 cup sugar

Add vinegar to dry mustard and stir until lumps disappear. Cover and let sit overnight.

Pour the mustard mixture into the top of a double boiler. Beat eggs, add sugar. Slowly add the egg and sugar mixture to the mustard. Cook over boiling water, stirring to avoid lumps for about 12 minutes until thickened. Pour into covered container and refrigerate. Keeps for months.

MILD MUSTARD

1 part Mayonnaise*
1 part Hot Mustard*

For those who prefer a milder mustard, mix equal parts mayonnaise with hot mustard recipe. Refrigerate.

Main Dish Sauces

EGG SAUCE FOR FISH

Serves 4

2 tablespoons pure
vegetable oil
2 tablespoons unbleached
flour
1 cup milk

½ teaspoon salt
¼ teaspoon dried minced
onion
Dash of pepper
1 hard-boiled egg, chopped

In a saucepan combine oil and flour and add milk. Stir constantly over medium heat until sauce boils. Add salt, onion, and pepper. Set aside and stir in chopped egg. Serve in gravy bowl so the sauce may be poured over the fish as needed.

TARTAR SAUCE

Makes 1 cup

1 cup Mayonnaise*
1 teaspoon grated onion
2 tablespoons capers,
slightly mashed

1 teaspoon minced parsley
¼ teaspoon dry mustard

Mix all ingredients thoroughly and chill. Serve over fish.

PARSLEY SAUCE

Makes 1 cup

2 cups chopped fresh
parsley leaves and
stems, washed and
drained
⅔ cup pure vegetable oil
⅔ cup grated Parmesan
cheese

1 teaspoon salt
½ teaspoon pepper
2 cloves garlic, minced
1 tablespoon dried sweet
basil (optional)

Combine all ingredients in blender until a smooth paste forms. Refrigerate in a covered container and use as needed. Use instead of Pesto Sauce* in making Pesto Pizza.*

To serve over hot spaghetti, rice, noodles, or potatoes, dilute with a little water and warm.

PESTO SAUCE

Makes ¾ cup

2 to 4 tablespoons dried
   sweet basil
2 cloves garlic
½ cup grated Parmesan
   cheese

1 teaspoon salt
1 teaspoon ground black
   pepper
½ cup pure vegetable oil

Combine all dry ingredients in a blender. Add half the vegetable oil. Blend on high speed. Add remaining oil and blend until thoroughly mixed.

If not used immediately, refrigerate in a covered container.

Pickles and Relishes

CORN RELISH

Makes 8 pints

12 full-size ears of corn
6 pounds (2 medium
   heads) cabbage
3 large green peppers
1 cup chopped
   celery or 1
   teaspoon celery seed
3 red peppers or 3 whole
   pimentos

4 onions
2 cups white distilled
   vinegar
2 cups water
2 tablespoons dry mustard
5 tablespoons salt
½ teaspoon turmeric
2 cups packed brown sugar

Cut corn off the cobs and place the kernels in large kettle. Chop cabbage, peppers, celery, red peppers, and onions and add to corn. Stir in all other ingredients and cook over medium heat until tender (about ½ hour). Then boil rapidly for 5 minutes. Pack in sterilized canning jars, leaving the relish about 1 inch below the top of the jar. Seal and process in boiling water bath for 15 minutes.

SPICED PEARS

Makes 3 pints

9 to 10 large firm pears
1½ cups white distilled
   vinegar
3 cups sugar

3 2-inch sticks whole
   cinnamon
1 whole nutmeg, cracked
   into large pieces

Peel, halve, and core pears. Combine vinegar and sugar in heavy saucepan. Wrap cinnamon and nutmeg in cheesecloth and add to vinegar and sugar mixture. Bring to a boil. Add pear halves and cook until tender. Pack pears in sterilized canning jars. Remove spices from vinegar solution and pour over pears, leaving ½ inch headspace. Seal. Process in boiling water bath for 15 minutes.

SWEET ZUCCHINI PICKLES

Makes 4 pints

8 cups sliced zucchini
4 cups water
¼ cup pickling lime
4 cups sugar
4 cups white distilled
   vinegar

1 2-inch stick cinnamon
1 whole nutmeg, cracked
   into large pieces
1 teaspoon celery seed
1 teaspoon salt

If zucchini has been waxed, peel before slicing. Soak sliced zucchini in water mixed with the pickling lime overnight. In the morning, drain, rinse several times in clear water, and let stand in clear cold water for 3 hours. Combine the remaining ingredients and bring to a boil. Pour the hot syrup over the drained zucchini slices and allow to stand overnight. When ready to pack, bring syrup to boil again. Remove cinnamon stick and nutmeg, and while hot, pack pickles and syrup into hot sterilized jars, leaving ½ inch headspace. Cap and process in boiling water bath for 10 minutes.

WATERMELON PICKLES

Makes 4 pints

8 cups cut-up watermelon
  rind
4 cups water
¼ cup pickling salt
4 cups sugar
2 cups white distilled
  vinegar

2 cups water
4 2-inch sticks cinnamon
2 whole nutmegs, cracked
  into pieces
¼ teaspoon mustard seed

Before measuring, peel the watermelon rind, cut off all pink portions, and cut into 1-inch chunks. Soak overnight in water mixed with the salt. In the morning drain and rinse several times with cold water. Place in a saucepan, cover with clear water, and boil until rind is tender. Drain. Combine sugar, vinegar, and water in pan. Tie the spices in a piece of cheesecloth and add to vinegar solution. Bring to a boil and continue to cook for 10 minutes. Remove from heat and allow to steep for an additional 15 minutes. Take the spices from the syrup, add drained watermelon rind, and cook until transparent. Pack rind into sterilized jars and pour syrup to cover rind, leaving ½ inch headspace. Cap, seal, and process in boiling water bath for 10 minutes.

ZUCCHINI DILL PICKLES

Makes 4 pints

2 quarts water
¾ cup pickling salt
8 cups zucchini (cut into
  long strips)
2 cups white distilled
  vinegar

2 cups water
6 cloves garlic
Dill seed
Mustard seed

In a large bowl combine water and ½ cup pickling salt. Place zucchini strips in the brine and allow to soak overnight. In the morning drain and rinse zucchini in clear cold water. In a saucepan combine vinegar, water, remaining ¼ cup salt, and garlic cloves. Bring to a boil. Remove from heat and allow to steep for about 15 minutes. Meanwhile, pack the zucchini tightly in sterilized canning jars. In each pint jar, put 2 tablespoons dill seed and 1 teaspoon mustard seed. Remove the garlic from the vinegar mixture and pour while hot over the zucchini strips, making sure the strips are completely covered and leaving ½ inch headspace. Seal jars tightly and process in a boiling water bath for 10 minutes.

Bread Crumbs and Croutons

DRY BREAD CRUMBS

Several slices stale bread

Oven 300°

Place stale bread on a cookie sheet and heat until dried. Put through blender, meat grinder, or place between two sheets of waxed paper and crush with a rolling pin. Place the crumbs in a covered container.

SOFT BREAD CRUMBS

Several slices 2- to 4-day-old bread

Bread may be broken up very lightly with your fingers or gently pulled apart using a fork. To retain the light texture, don't crush the bread when preparing the crumbs. When measuring soft bread crumbs, pile them lightly into a measuring cup without packing them down.

CHEESY CROUTONS

Several slices day-old bread
Uncolored butter
Parmesan cheese, grated

Oven 375°

Butter slices of bread and sprinkle them well with Parmesan cheese. Cut bread into cubes and brown in oven, about 15 minutes.

CROUTONS ITALIANO

Makes 4 cups

4 cups bread cubes
2 teaspoons Italian herb
  seasoning

½ teaspoon garlic salt
½ cup uncolored butter,
  melted

Oven 350°

Place cubes in a 12×8×2-inch baking dish (or equivalent) and bake in oven until cubes begin to dry, about 10 minutes. Sprinkle herb seasoning and garlic salt evenly over the cubes. Drizzle with melted butter and toss to coat all cubes. Return to oven for 30 to 45 minutes, stirring every 10 minutes until croutons are very crisp and dry. Cool and store in a tightly covered container.

Stocks

BEEF STOCK

Makes 1 quart

6 pounds beef soup bones
  or 2 pounds cheap cut
  of beef
2½ quarts cold water
1 cup sliced onions
½ cup chopped celery with
  leaves

1 bay leaf
Several sprigs parsley or
  dried flakes
2 teaspoons salt
Pepper, as desired

In a large pot or Dutch oven cover beef and/or beef bones with cold water. Bring to a boil, add rest of ingredients, and simmer covered for 2 hours. Strain. Remove meat from bones and store in refrigerator for further use. Refrigerate broth. When ready to use, skim off fat and reheat.

CHICKEN STOCK

Makes 2 quarts

4 pounds (about) chicken
   bones or whole carcass,
   broken up
4 quarts cold water
1 medium onion, diced, or
   instant minced onion

1 carrot, diced
Several stalks celery, diced
Salt and pepper to taste

Cover chicken bones with cold water in a Dutch oven. Add onion, carrot, and celery and bring slowly to a boil. Simmer for 2 to 3 hours. Strain, season, and cool. Refrigerate. Skim off layer of fat on top when ready to use stock.

Dessert Sauces and Syrups

BUTTERSCOTCH SAUCE

Makes 1 cup

1 egg yolk, slightly beaten
¼ cup uncolored butter
¼ cup milk

⅔ cup packed brown sugar
⅓ cup light corn syrup
⅛ teaspoon salt

Mix all ingredients in a heavy saucepan. Cook over low heat, stirring constantly until thick, about 12 to 15 minutes. Use immediately or cool and refrigerate in a covered container. Serve cold or reheat in a double boiler.

CAROB OR CHOCOLATE SYRUP

Makes 2 cups

A thin syrup good for making milk shakes, sodas, or as a sauce for ice cream.

1 cup sugar
½ cup carob powder or
  dry cocoa
¼ teaspoon salt

1 cup milk
2 teaspoons pure vanilla
  extract

Combine sugar, carob powder, and salt in a saucepan. Add milk and stir until smooth. Bring to a boil, stirring constantly over medium heat. Reduce heat and continue cooking for 1 minute.

Remove pan from heat and add vanilla. Cool to room temperature and refrigerate for future use.

FUDGE SAUCE

Makes 1¾ cups

¾ cup cocoa
1 cup sugar
¼ teaspoon salt
⅔ cup milk
¼ cup light corn syrup

2 tablespoons uncolored
  butter
1 teaspoon pure vanilla
  extract

Combine cocoa, sugar, and salt in a medium saucepan. Slowly stir in milk and corn syrup and mix until smooth. Bring to a boil over medium heat, stirring constantly. Cook over low heat, stirring frequently, for 5 to 7 minutes until very thick. Remove from heat and stir in butter and vanilla. Let cool and refrigerate in covered container. Serve cold or reheat in a double boiler.

LEMON SAUCE FOR GINGERBREAD

Makes 1 cup

1 tablespoon cornstarch
½ cup sugar
1 cup water
1 tablespoon pure
   vegetable oil or
   uncolored butter

⅛ teaspoon salt
2 tablespoons pure lemon
   juice

In a saucepan, mix cornstarch and sugar and slowly stir in water. Bring to a boil over medium heat. Stir constantly. When sauce starts to boil continue stirring and boil for 1 minute. Remove from heat. Add oil or butter, salt, and lemon juice. Mix well. Serve warm over gingerbread.

MARSHMALLOW SAUCE

Makes 4 cups

2 envelopes unflavored
   gelatin
½ cup cold water
2 cups sugar
¾ cup boiling water

½ teaspoon salt
1½ teaspoons pure vanilla
   extract
½ cup milk

Soften gelatin in cold water. In a 2-quart heavy saucepan add sugar to boiling water. Continue boiling until syrup reaches the thread stage (230–234°) or thread forms when syrup is dropped from the edge of a spoon. Remove from heat.

Add softened gelatin to hot syrup and stir until dissolved. Cool 10 to 15 minutes. Add salt and vanilla. Beat with mixer until mixture becomes thick and cool. Add cold milk and continue beating until fluffy. Serve over ice cream.

Store sauce in a covered container in the refrigerator. If sauce is too thick, it may be thinned by adding more milk to the sauce in the top of double boiler and beating until fluffy and creamy.

MAPLE SYRUP I

Makes 3 cups

8-ounce bottle pure maple syrup
2 cups light corn syrup

Combine pure maple syrup and corn syrup and use as a topping for pancakes and waffles.

MAPLE SYRUP II

Makes 1 cup

½ cup water
1 cup packed brown sugar
1 tablespoon uncolored
   butter

3 tablespoons pure maple
   syrup

In a saucepan combine water and brown sugar. Heat over medium heat until sugar is dissolved. Add butter and maple syrup and heat several more minutes. Use immediately or refrigerate in a covered container. Reheat before using.

PINEAPPLE SYRUP

Makes 2 cups

1 20-ounce can unsweetened crushed pineapple
¾ cup sugar

Place undrained pineapple in blender on highest speed until smooth. Pour into a heavy saucepan. Stir in sugar. Bring to a boil, stirring frequently. Cool. Refrigerate in a covered container. Use as needed for pineapple milk shakes, sodas, popsicles, or as a topping for ice cream.

WHIPPED TOPPING

Makes 3 cups

½ teaspoon unflavored
  gelatin
¼ cup cold water
½ cup evaporated milk

1 teaspoon pure vanilla
  extract
1 tablespoon sugar

Soften gelatin in cold water. In a small saucepan heat milk over medium heat. Add softened gelatin and stir until completely dissolved. Pour milk into a shallow bowl and chill for 2 hours. Place mixing bowl in refrigerator to chill. Whip milk in chilled bowl until it holds its shape. Add vanilla and sugar and continue beating until well mixed. Refrigerate covered until ready to use.

Jams and Jellies

CRANBERRY JELLY OR SAUCE

Makes 1 quart

1 pound cranberries, fresh or frozen (thawed), washed
  thoroughly
2 cups boiling water
2 cups sugar

In a large saucepan combine berries and boiling water. When water comes to the boil again, cover the saucepan. Cook cranberries for 4 minutes or until the skins burst. Put the berries through a food mill or press firmly through a strainer. Add sugar. Bring mixture to a full boil. Cranberry sauce requires no further cooking. Cover and refrigerate.

A molded cranberry jelly needs continuous boiling and stirring for 5 minutes longer. Pour into a wet 1½-quart mold. Cover and refrigerate.

BLUEBERRY-PINEAPPLE JAM

Makes 2 cups

2 cups fresh or frozen (thawed) blueberries
1 cup finely chopped fresh pineapple
2½ cups sugar

Combine fruit and sugar in a heavy saucepan. Slowly bring to a boil, stirring until sugar dissolves. Whir in a blender until large lumps disappear.

Return mixture to stove, cooking rapidly until thick. As mixture thickens, stir frequently. Pour mixture boiling hot into sterilized canning jars. Seal. Or cool and refrigerate in a covered container and use as needed.

BLUEBERRY JAM

Makes 1 cup

2 cups fresh or frozen (thawed) blueberries
1⅓ cups sugar

Mash blueberries in the bottom of a heavy saucepan. Add sugar and mix well. Bring slowly to boiling, stirring occasionally until sugar dissolves. Continue boiling rapidly until jam thickens. As jam thickens, stir frequently to prevent sticking. Pour boiling hot into sterilized canning jars. Seal. Or cool and refrigerate in a covered container.

PEAR JAM

Makes 1 cup

2 cups peeled, sliced pears   ½ to 1 cup sugar
¼ cup water
2 tablespoons pure lemon
   juice

Combine all ingredients in a heavy saucepan. Cook over medium heat until pears are tender. Place in blender on medium speed for several seconds until desired consistency is reached. Return to saucepan and continue cooking over medium heat for about 20 minutes or until jam thickens. Pour boiling hot into sterilized canning jars. Seal. Or cool and refrigerate in a covered container.

PINEAPPLE JAM

Makes 1 cup

2 cups finely chopped fresh
  pineapple
½ cup water

1 cup sugar
2 teaspoons pure lemon
  juice

Combine all ingredients in a heavy saucepan. Slowly bring to boiling, stirring occasionally until sugar dissolves. Cook rapidly until thick, about 30 minutes. As jam thickens, stir frequently to prevent sticking. Pour boiling hot into sterilized canning jars. Seal. Or cool and refrigerate in a covered container.

RHUBARB JAM

Makes 2 cups

1½ cups sugar
½ cup water
1 pound rhubarb, fresh or
  frozen (thawed), cut up

2 teaspoons pure lemon
  juice

In a heavy saucepan over high heat, dissolve sugar in water, stirring until mixture boils. Add rhubarb. Cool. Place in blender on high speed for a few seconds until desired consistency is reached.

Return mixture to saucepan and add lemon juice. Cook over high heat until jam thickens. Pour boiling hot into sterilized canning jars. Seal. Or cool and refrigerate in a covered container.

BLUEBERRY-RHUBARB JAM

Makes 2 cups

2 cups blueberries, fresh,
canned, or frozen
(thawed)
2 cups cut-up rhubarb,
fresh or frozen
(thawed)

½ cup water
1 cup sugar
2 tablespoons pure lemon
juice

Combine all ingredients in a large, heavy saucepan. Cook over medium heat until fruit is tender. Cool. Place in blender on medium speed for several seconds until desired consistency is reached. Return to saucepan and continue cooking over medium heat until jam thickens, about 30 to 45 minutes. Stir occasionally. Pour boiling hot into sterilized canning jars. Seal. Or cool and refrigerate in a covered container.

PAPAYA AND PINEAPPLE JAM

Makes 4 cups

1 20-ounce can crushed
pineapple in heavy syrup
3 cups chopped peeled
papayas (about 2 6-inch
papayas)

1 cup sugar
1 teaspoon ground ginger
(optional)
¼ cup pure lemon juice

Pour pineapple with its syrup into blender. Add chopped papayas. Blend for several seconds until fruit has the desired consistency.

Pour fruits into a heavy saucepan. Add sugar, ginger, and lemon juice. Bring to a boil, stirring frequently. Simmer jam until it thickens, about 20 to 30 minutes. Pour boiling hot into sterilized canning jars. Seal. Or cool and refrigerate in a covered container.

ZUCCHINI AND PINEAPPLE JAM

Makes 2½ cups

4 cups (about 2 pounds)
   peeled and thinly sliced
   zucchini
¼ cup pure lemon juice
¼ teaspoon pure lemon
   extract

1 13½-ounce can (2 cups)
   sweetened crushed
   pineapple, drained
2 cups sugar

Place all ingredients in a large, heavy saucepan. Bring to a boil, then simmer 15 to 30 minutes, stirring occasionally, until zucchini is tender and mixture finally thickens. Pour boiling hot into sterilized canning jars. Seal. Or cool and refrigerate in a covered container.

Food Colorings

BLUE COLORING

Makes about 1½ cups

1 cup water
1 cup blueberries

Boil water and blueberries slowly for about 5 minutes. Strain well, reserving the liquid. A few drops will color icing bluish-purple and, of course, the taste is delicious.

To dye eggs, add 1 tablespoon white distilled vinegar to 1 cup of blueberry coloring. Eggs turn a pretty bluish-lavender color.

BROWN COLORING

Makes 1 cup

1 cup brewed coffee

One cup of coffee with 2 tablespoons vinegar added will dye eggs brown.

Use carob powder, cocoa, or chocolate to color icing brown.

GREEN COLORING

Alfalfa tea

Alfalfa tea may be purchased at health food stores if you can't find it elsewhere. It will not work as an egg dye, but small amounts can be added to icing to make it green. However, the icing does taste like grass so you may wish to limit its use to small amounts for leaves or other trimming.

PEACH COLORING

1 part Yellow Coloring*
1 part canned beet juice

This combination turns icing a pretty peach color. Likewise, when eggs are submerged in the solution with 1 tablespoon white distilled vinegar added, they also turn a pretty peach color.

PINK COLORING

Cranberry juice cocktail

Substitute cranberry juice cocktail for liquid in icing recipe. Adds a delicious flavor.

RED COLORING

Makes 1½ cups

3 fresh beets, washed and diced
1½ cups water

Slowly boil beets in water for about 5 minutes. Let stand until cool. Strain, discarding solid residue. For red icing, substitute the beet juice for some of the liquid. The icing picks up little of the beet flavor.

To dye eggs, add 1 tablespoon white distilled vinegar to 1 cup beet juice. Will dye shell pink-red, depending on length of time egg is submerged.

YELLOW COLORING

1 teaspoon saffron
1 cup water

Saffron can be found in the spice section of many supermarkets. It's expensive but a little goes a long way. Add the saffron to water and boil slowly for about 5 minutes. Let stand until cool. Strain well.

Add a few drops of the coloring to icing for a pretty yellow color. The sweetness of the icing counteracts the bitterness of the saffron.

For egg dye, add 1 tablespoon white distilled vinegar to 1 cup of yellow coloring and submerge egg. Will dye the egg bright yellow.

YELLOW/ORANGE COLORING

One carrot and ¼ cup water or canned carrot juice

Wash carrot well and cut into pieces skin and all. Place in blender with water on high speed until smooth. Add small amounts of the paste to icing to color it orange.

Carrot juice may be used to color icing yellow or orange. Decrease liquid in icing recipe slightly and substitute carrot juice. Carrot paste or juice will not dye eggs, however.

Miscellaneous

CAROB POWDER

Carob flour

Oven 300°

If you buy carob in flour form, you can make it into powder by toasting it in the oven. Spread the flour in a thin layer on a cookie sheet and toast for about 15 minutes or until the color of cocoa (light brown).

A general rule in using carob powder as a substitute for chocolate is 3 tablespoons of carob powder or cocoa equals one square of unsweetened chocolate.

HOMEMADE PAPAYA CONCENTRATE

Makes 2 cups

If you can't find prepared papaya concentrate at your local store, you can make your own. The following proportions will differ depending on the size of papayas available.

2 fresh papayas (each   ¼ cup pure lemon juice
    about 6 inches long)   1 cup water
½ cup sugar

Peel papayas and remove all seeds. Cut into several pieces and place in a large saucepan. Cover with sugar. Let stand about 15 minutes. Place in blender on high speed for several seconds. Add lemon juice and water. Bring mixture to a boil and continue boiling for several minutes. Chill. Use for Papaya Gelatin.*

Like fresh pineapples, papayas contain an enzyme that will keep gelatin from congealing unless the enzyme is destroyed by heat first.

SOY EGG YOLK SUBSTITUTE

Makes 2 to 2½ cups

When eggs are used for binding purposes as in cookies, meat loaf, muffins, etc., this may be used as a substitute if your child is allergic to eggs or seems to get a hyperactive reaction.

1 cup soy powder or soy
  flour
2 cups water

2 tablespoons pure
  vegetable oil
¼ teaspoon salt

Thoroughly blend powder and water in a blender at high speed. Pour into the top of a double boiler and cook over boiling water, covered, for about 1 hour. Beat in oil and salt with an electric mixer. Refrigerate. Will thicken when cooled.

Use about ¼ cup of the substitute for each egg. Will not act as a leavening agent as eggs do in some recipes.

3

Basic Breads

You may or may not decide to make your own breads. There are several brands of "safe" frozen bread doughs available (see Appendix B). From these basic doughs you can make many other bread products like doughnuts or sweet rolls. There are also several brands of baked goods available that appear to be okay. Check labels to be sure products contain no bleached flour, artificial colors, flavorings, or preservatives.

On the other hand, if you make your own bread products you will know precisely what ingredients are used, a definite advantage when you're searching for clues as to what is bothering your child. The recipes we've included are all easily prepared. We especially recommend both the yeast and baking powder batter breads. They're easier to make than the kneaded breads and taste delicious. You don't have to be a slave to your dough while you're waiting for it to rise. If you wish to delay the rising action, place the dough in the refrigerator. If the dough rises too much, punch it down and let it rise again. Even if your loaves don't look beautiful, your child won't care and the homemade taste is irresistible.

Remember to avoid the following in choosing your ingredients:

> Bleached white flour
> Yeast with BHA/BHT
> Colored butter or margarine
> Raisins
> Almonds

WHITE BREAD

Makes 2 loaves

2 cups milk
2 packages dry yeast or 2
    cakes compressed yeast
¼ cup warm water
2 tablespoons sugar

1 tablespoon salt
¼ cup pure vegetable oil
    or ¼ cup uncolored
    butter, melted
6–7 cups unbleached flour

Oven 400°

Scald milk and allow to cool to room temperature. Dissolve yeast in warm water. Add sugar. Let stand until yeast mixture starts to bubble. Add salt, oil or butter, and about half the flour to cooled milk. Beat with an electric mixer on medium speed for about 2 minutes. Add yeast mixture and beat well. Slowly stir in remaining flour with a heavy spoon. Place on floured surface and knead until dough is smooth and elastic, about 10 minutes.

Place dough in a greased bowl, turning to grease the top too. Cover. Let rise in a warm place until double in bulk, about 1 or 2 hours. Punch dough down. Let dough rise again until double in bulk, about 1 hour. Place on lightly floured surface. Divide dough into two parts. Cover with cloth and let rest about 15 minutes. Make into 2 loaves and place in 2 greased 9×5-inch loaf pans. Cover and let rise until double in bulk, about ½ hour. Bake for 50 minutes. Remove from pans. If bottom of loaves sound hollow when tapped, bread is done. Cool on wire racks.

HIGH PROTEIN BREAD

Makes 2 loaves

Dry milk, soy flour, and eggs add extra nutrition to this tasty bread.

2 packages dry yeast or 2
cakes compressed yeast
⅔ cup warm water
1 tablespoon dark brown
sugar
1 cup instant dry milk
¼ cup dark brown sugar
or molasses

2 teaspoons salt
1¾ cups warm water
5½ to 6½ cups whole
wheat flour
2 eggs, room temperature
¼ cup pure vegetable oil
1 cup soy flour

Oven 400°

Dissolve yeast in ⅔ cup warm water. Add 1 tablespoon sugar and stir. Set aside for 10 minutes. In the meantime, add dry milk, sugar or molasses, and salt to 1¾ cups warm water. Stir until dissolved. In a large bowl, add yeast mixture to milk mixture. Add 3 cups whole wheat flour and stir well, using wooden spoon. Beat at least 300 strokes by hand or beat with an electric mixer for 10 minutes. Add eggs and oil and mix thoroughly.

Add enough of remaining flour (whole wheat and soy) to make a kneadable dough. Turn dough out on lightly floured surface. Cover and let rest 20 minutes. Knead for 10 minutes or until dough is smooth and elastic. Place dough in an oiled 4-quart bowl. Turn completely over so that top is oiled. Place in a warm location until double in bulk, about 1 hour. Punch down. Divide into two portions. Cover and let rest 10 minutes. With a rolling pin, roll each portion into a 9×14-inch rectangle. Roll dough tightly into a cylinder. Pinch seam to seal. Place in well-greased 9×5-inch loaf pans. Let rise in warm place until double in bulk, about 1 hour. Bake at 400° for 10 minutes. Reduce heat to 350° and bake 40 more minutes. When done, remove from pans immediately and cool on wire racks. Brush top of hot loaves with uncolored butter for tender crust.

RYE BREAD

Makes 2 loaves

2 packages dry yeast or 2
   cakes compressed yeast
1¾ cups warm water
⅓ cup honey
1 tablespoon salt
2 tablespoons pure
   vegetable oil

1 tablespoon caraway seed
3 cups sifted rye flour
1½ to 2 cups unbleached
   sifted flour

Oven 400°

Dissolve yeast in warm water. Add honey, salt, and oil. Add caraway seed and 2 cups rye flour. Beat with mixer until very smooth. With a heavy spoon, stir in the rest of the rye flour and enough white flour to make dough leave sides of the bowl. Turn dough out onto a lightly floured board and knead gently until smooth and elastic, adding flour when necessary. Place dough in a greased bowl and turn greased side to the top. Cover and allow to rise in a warm place until double in bulk, about 1 hour. Punch down and shape into two loaves. Place in greased loaf pans, cover and allow to rise again until 1 inch above tops of pans. Bake 30 to 35 minutes. Remove from pans. If bottoms of loaves sound hollow when tapped, bread is done. Place on wire racks, spread tops lightly with uncolored butter, and allow to cool.

NO-KNEAD WHITE BATTER BREAD

Makes 2 loaves

This is our favorite quick, easily prepared white bread. Requires no kneading and only one rising. Flavor is good and it makes great toast. Does not have as nice a texture as kneaded bread.

2 cups milk
½ cup pure vegetable oil
   or melted uncolored
   butter
2 teaspoons salt
3 packages dry yeast or 3
   cakes compressed yeast

1 cup warm water
¼ cup sugar
5 to 5½ cups unsifted
   unbleached flour

Oven 400°

Scald milk. Add shortening and salt. Cool to lukewarm. Dissolve yeast in warm water. Add sugar. Let sit until bubbly. Combine milk and yeast mixtures in large mixing bowl. Add half the flour. Beat for several minutes with an electric mixer. Work in remaining flour. Pour into two well-greased 9×5-inch loaf pans. Cover. Let rise in warm place until double in bulk—about 30 to 45 minutes. Bake for 1 hour. Remove from pans. If bottoms of loaves sound hollow when tapped, bread is done. Cool on wire racks. May be well wrapped and frozen.

NO-KNEAD WHOLE WHEAT BATTER BREAD

Makes 2 loaves

½ cup uncolored butter,
   melted
2 cups milk, scalded
¼ cup honey
1 tablespoon salt
3 packages dry yeast or 3
   cakes compressed yeast

1 cup warm water
3 cups whole wheat flour
2½ to 2¾ cups
   unbleached white flour

Oven 400°

Combine butter, milk, honey, and salt and cool until lukewarm. Dissolve yeast in warm water. Set aside for 10 minutes. Add to milk mixture. Stir in whole wheat flour and part of the white flour. Beat with an electric mixer for 2 minutes. Add remaining white flour and stir well, using a heavy spoon. Pour into two well-greased 9×5-inch loaf pans. Cover and let rise in a warm place for about 45 minutes or until double in bulk. Bake for 1 hour. Remove from pans. If bottoms of loaves sound hollow when tapped, bread is done. Lightly spread uncolored butter on tops of loaves for a softer crust. Let loaves cool thoroughly on a wire rack.

NO-KNEAD WHITE REFRIGERATOR ROLLS

Makes 3 to 4 dozen rolls

A family favorite, easy to prepare, and can be baked as needed.

2 cups milk, scalded
2 packages dry yeast or 2
   cakes compressed yeast
½ cup sugar

2 teaspoons salt
⅓ cup pure vegetable oil
6 to 6½ cups unsifted un-
   bleached flour

Oven 400°

Scald milk. Cool to lukewarm. Dissolve yeast in milk. Add sugar, salt, and oil. Add half the flour and beat with an electric mixer for 2 minutes. Gradually add remaining flour and continue beating until dough is smooth. Cover with a damp cloth, placing waxed paper or foil over the cloth to keep the moisture in. Refrigerate. Dough will keep for several days and can be used any time. If any dough remains after about 4 days, make it up into rolls that can be served immediately or frozen for future use.

To bake rolls, remove desired amount of dough from refrigerator several hours prior to baking. With floured hands, pat the dough out on a floured surface and cut out rolls with a round cookie cutter. Fold one half of each circle over onto itself and place on a greased baking sheet or pan. Place rolls so that they are just touching each other. Cover with a cloth and let rise in a warm place for about 1½ hours. Bake about 15 minutes, depending on the size of the rolls. Remove from pan and serve warm.

NO-KNEAD WHOLE WHEAT REFRIGERATOR ROLLS

Makes 2 dozen rolls

2 packages dry yeast or 2 cakes compressed yeast
2 cups warm water
⅓ cup packed brown sugar
2 tablespoons honey
2 teaspoons salt

¼ cup pure vegetable oil
2 cups whole wheat flour
2¼ to 2½ cups unbleached unsifted flour

Oven 400°

Dissolve yeast in warm water. Stir in brown sugar and honey. Let sit 10 minutes. Add salt and oil. Stir in whole wheat flour. Beat with an electric mixer for 2 minutes. Stir in unbleached flour. Mix well. Cover dough with a damp cloth. Refrigerate for up to several days. Punch dough down as needed.

When ready to bake rolls, remove dough from refrigerator. With floured hands, pinch off pieces of dough of desired size. Form into balls and place close together on a well-greased pan. Cover with a cloth and let rise in a warm place until almost double in bulk, 30 to 45 minutes. Bake for 15 minutes or until rolls are lightly browned on the bottom. Remove all rolls from pan and serve. Leftovers may be frozen and reheated.

ENGLISH MUFFINS

Makes about 20 3-inch rounds

1 package dry active yeast or 1 cake compressed yeast
¼ cup warm water
2 tablespoons sugar
1 cup milk
½ cup water

3 tablespoons pure vegetable oil
2 teaspoons salt
4 to 4½ cups unsifted unbleached flour
Corn meal

Dissolve yeast in warm water. Add sugar. Set aside. Scald milk. Add water, oil, and salt. Let cool. When lukewarm, add about half the flour and mix well. Stir in yeast mixture. Gradually beat in remaining flour to form a moderately stiff dough. Place in a greased bowl, turning to grease top too. Cover with a damp cloth. Let rise in a warm place until dough doubles in bulk, about 1 to 1½ hours. Place on a lightly floured surface and knead about 1 minute.

Roll out dough until ¼ inch thick. Cut circles of desired size with cookie cutters, sharp tin cans, or doughnut cutter without the hole. Sprinkle a little corn meal on both sides of each muffin. Let stand in a warm place about 15 minutes or until they begin to rise.

Lightly grease a heavy skillet or griddle. Preheat stove top or griddle to medium heat. Place muffins on hot surface. Turn when browned. Total cooking time is about 8 to 10 minutes. Serve hot or let cool. Cut in half and toast. Or freeze muffins in plastic bags and remove as needed. Delicious warm with butter and honey or jam.

PITA POCKET BREAD

Makes about 20 4-inch rounds

Kids really enjoy these tasty, chewy individual "loaves" with a hollow pocket inside, just right for their favorite filling.

2 packages dry yeast or 2
    cakes compressed yeast
2½ cups warm water
1 teaspoon sugar
1½ tablespoons salt

1 tablespoon pure
    vegetable oil
5 to 6 cups unbleached
    flour

Oven 500°

Dissolve yeast in water. Add sugar, salt, oil. Using an electric mixer, add half the flour and beat well. Gradually add more flour until dough is sticky. Work in remaining flour and knead dough for 5 to 10 minutes until smooth and elastic. Divide dough into about twenty pieces (fewer if you desire larger loaves). Let rise for about 2 hours.

Place rounds on ungreased cookie sheet. If your oven will hold two sheets on one oven rack, you may bake them together. Otherwise, bake only one sheet at a time. Place cookie sheet on lowest rack of the oven. Bake for 5 minutes undisturbed. Then move sheet to higher shelf and bake loaves until puffy and lightly browned, about 3 to 5 minutes.

Immediately wrap hot loaves well in foil or plastic bags to prevent crispness and ensure a chewy, spongy texture. As the loaves cool, they will lose their puffy appearance. When cool, slit one side and fill the pocket with seasoned hamburger, egg salad, Tomato-less Chili,* etc. Loaves may be frozen for future use.

SANDWICH BUNS

Makes 18 buns

4½ to 5 cups unbleached
   flour
1 package dry yeast or 1
   cake compressed yeast
2 cups water

2 tablespoons sugar
2 tablespoons pure
   vegetable oil
2 teaspoons salt

Oven 350°

In a large mixing bowl combine 2 cups flour and yeast. In a saucepan mix water, sugar, oil, and salt. Heat until warm, stirring constantly. Add to dry ingredients and beat with mixer at low speed until blended. Mix at high speed for 3 minutes. Stir in by hand enough of the remaining flour to make a fairly stiff dough. Turn out onto a floured board and knead for about 10 minutes or until smooth and elastic. Place in a greased bowl and turn over dough so top is greased. Cover and let rise in a warm place until double in bulk, about 1½ hours. Punch down and let dough rest for 10 minutes. Roll out so dough is ½ inch thick and cut into 3-inch rounds with a floured cutter. Place on a greased cookie sheet, cover, and let rise until double in bulk, about 1 hour. Bake for 20 to 25 minutes or until lightly browned. While still warm from the oven, brush tops lightly with uncolored butter.

BANANA BREAD (EGGLESS)

Makes 1 loaf

1¾ cups sifted unbleached flour
1½ teaspoons baking powder
½ teaspoon baking soda
¾ teaspoon salt

⅓ cup pure vegetable oil
⅔ cup sugar
¼ cup water
1 cup (2 or 3 bananas) mashed bananas
½ cup finely chopped nuts

Oven 350°

In a small bowl mix sifted flour, baking powder, baking soda, and salt. Set aside. In a large bowl beat together on low speed oil, sugar, and water. Gradually add flour mixture alternately with mashed bananas until all ingredients are well blended. Stir in chopped nuts. Pour into a greased 9×5-inch loaf pan and bake for 1 hour, or until a toothpick inserted in the middle comes out clean. Cool in pan for 15 minutes. Turn out onto wire rack and cool completely. Wrap and store in refrigerator.

CRANBERRY BREAD

Makes 1 loaf

2 cups sifted unbleached flour
1¼ cups sugar
1½ teaspoons baking powder
1 teaspoon salt
½ teaspoon baking soda
½ teaspoon nutmeg

¼ cup pure vegetable oil
¼ cup pure lemon juice and pulp
1 egg, well beaten
1 cup coarsely chopped cranberries
½ cup chopped nuts
½ cup chopped dates

Oven 350°

Combine all dry ingredients and mix well. Stir in oil, lemon juice, and egg, mixing batter well after each addition. Fold in cranberries, nuts, and dates. Pour into a well-greased 9×5×3-inch loaf pan. Bake for 1 hour or until a toothpick inserted in the center comes out clean. Cool in the pan for 20 minutes. Turn out onto wire rack and cool. Refrigerate for 24 hours before serving for best results. Makes great-tasting toast.

DATE AND NUT BREAD

Makes 1 loaf

1 cup chopped dates
¾ cup boiling water
1½ cups sifted unbleached
   flour
2 teaspoons baking powder
½ teaspoon salt
3 tablespoons pure
   vegetable oil

¾ cup firmly packed
   brown sugar
2 eggs, slightly beaten
1 teaspoon pure vanilla
   extract
¾ cup chopped walnuts

Oven 350°

In a small bowl soak dates in boiling water. Place in refrigerator to cool. In a small bowl combine flour, baking powder, and salt. Set aside. In a large bowl beat together oil, brown sugar, eggs, and vanilla. Gradually add flour mixture alternately with soaked dates and water until mixture is well blended. Stir in chopped walnuts. Pour into a greased 9×5-inch loaf pan. Bake for 1 hour or until toothpick inserted in the middle comes out clean. Cool in pan for 15 minutes. Turn out onto wire rack. Cool completely. Wrap in foil and refrigerate.

PUMPKIN BREAD

Makes 2 loaves

3 cups unsifted unbleached
   flour
1½ cups sugar
1 teaspoon cinnamon
1 teaspoon salt
¾ teaspoon nutmeg
2 teaspoons baking soda
½ teaspoon baking powder

1½ cups canned or cooked
   pumpkin
¾ cup milk
½ cup pure vegetable oil
2 eggs, slightly beaten
1 cup chopped nuts
½ cup wheat germ
   (optional)

Oven 350°

Combine all ingredients in a large mixing bowl. Mix until just blended. Pour batter into two greased 9×5×3-inch loaf pans. Bake 50 to 60 minutes or until a toothpick inserted in the center comes out clean. Cool in pans for 10 minutes. Turn out onto wire racks. Cool completely.

ZUCCHINI BREAD

Makes 2 loaves

A family favorite.

3 eggs
1 cup pure vegetable oil
2 cups sugar
2 cups chopped zucchini, peeled (if zucchini is waxed) or unpeeled
3 cups unbleached flour

1 teaspoon baking soda
1 teaspoon salt
½ teaspoon nutmeg
1 teaspoon cinnamon
1 tablespoon pure vanilla extract
½ cup chopped nuts

Oven 350°

Mix together eggs, oil, and sugar. Add chopped zucchini to this mixture in a blender or beat in a large mixing bowl with electric mixer. Add flour, soda, salt, nutmeg, cinnamon, vanilla, and chopped nuts. Pour into two 9×5×3-inch greased loaf pans. Bake for 1 hour. Let cool 10 minutes. Remove from pan. Cool completely.

Eggless Zucchini Bread: Omit the eggs in the above recipe. Add 6 tablespoons water. Bake as above.

CAKE DOUGHNUTS

Makes 2½ dozen doughnuts

3 eggs
1 cup sugar
2 tablespoons uncolored
   butter, softened
1 cup mashed potatoes
3 cups unbleached flour

1 tablespoon baking
   powder
1 teaspoon salt
½ teaspoon cinnamon
¼ teaspoon nutmeg

In a large mixing bowl beat eggs until very light and fluffy. Add sugar and butter and continue to beat until very light. Blend in mashed potatoes. In a separate bowl combine the dry ingredients. Slowly add to the egg mixture, beating on low speed. When the flour mixture has been evenly mixed in, turn out the dough onto a floured board. Knead gently, using only enough additional flour to keep it from sticking to the board. Roll out the dough to ⅓-inch thickness and cut with a floured doughnut cutter. Deep fry both doughnuts and holes at 370° until golden brown on both sides. Coat lightly with sugar while still warm.

YEAST DOUGHNUTS

Makes 18 doughnuts

1 package dry yeast or 1
   cake compressed yeast
¼ cup warm water
3 tablespoons uncolored
   butter
1 cup milk, scalded

½ cup sugar
1 teaspoon salt
1 egg, beaten
3½ to 4 cups sifted
   unbleached flour

Sprinkle yeast over warm water and allow to dissolve. Add butter to scalded milk and stir until butter is melted. When milk is lukewarm, stir in yeast, sugar, salt, and egg. Mix thoroughly. Stir in 2 cups flour and beat with mixer until very smooth. With heavy spoon stir in enough flour so that dough leaves sides of the bowl. Turn dough out on a lightly floured board and knead until dough is smooth and elastic, adding flour if necessary. Place dough in greased bowl, turning greased side to the top. Cover and put in a warm place until double in bulk, about 1 hour. Punch down dough and turn out on board. Roll dough out to ⅓-inch thickness. Cut with floured doughnut cutter and place on cookie sheet. Knead scraps together slightly and reroll to cut more doughnuts. Cover doughnuts and allow to rise until almost double in bulk, about 1 hour. Fry in oil at 370° until golden brown on both sides. Coat with granulated or confectioners' sugar.

Doughnut Glaze: 1 cup confectioners' sugar together with just enough milk to make a slightly runny icing. Dip doughnuts in glaze. Serve warm or cold.

4

Breakfast: Getting a Good Start to the Day

Your child needs a good nutritious breakfast to start his day. It doesn't have to require a lot of preparation time nor does it have to be a large meal. You'll know best what kind of breakfast will appeal to your child.

Most kids really miss the forbidden additive-filled cereals and orange juice or prepared breakfast drinks. However, there are both hot and cold cereals available that are additive-free. If your child likes eggs, he can have these prepared as he desires. But no bacon or ham in any form for now. You can substitute homemade pork sausage or goetta. Store-bought sweet rolls are mostly taboo but you can easily make your own in quantity and freeze them for future use. Non-salicylate fruits and their juices should be encouraged, especially those rich in vitamin C—grapefruit, pineapple, and cranberry juice cocktail. Bananas are also nutritious, satisfying, and liked by many kids.

If your child isn't wild about breakfast, try serving some non-breakfast-type foods—hamburgers, fruit gelatin, French fries or hash browns, peanut butter and jelly (homemade) sandwiches or grilled cheese sandwiches.

In preparing breakfasts remember to avoid the following:

Artificially colored or flavored cereals, drinks, or breads
Colored butter
Salicylate fruits and fruit drinks—oranges, apples, etc.
Ham or bacon
Bleached white flour

BREAKFAST FRUIT PIZZA

Makes 8 individual pizzas

These breakfast pizzas make a tasty, nutritious start to the day. They may be made ahead of time and reheated. They are also great snacks or desserts.

1 recipe Pizza Crust*

Blueberry Filling

4 cups blueberries	16 ounces cream cheese,
¼ cup water	softened (optional)
½ cup sugar	Mozzarella cheese, grated
½ cup flour	or sliced

Oven 450°

Prepare pizza crust. While dough is rising, prepare filling. Put blueberries in a saucepan. Add water and sugar. Heat until sugar is dissolved and blueberries are tender. Add flour and cook until mixture thickens. Remove from heat.

Divide dough into eight portions. Roll out each and place on oiled cookie sheet or pizza pan. Turn up the edges of each. Spread each with cream cheese, if desired. Add blueberry filling. Bake for 15 minutes. Top with mozzarella cheese and return to oven for another 5 to 10 minutes or until crust is browned. Serve hot.

Pizzas may also be prepared ahead of time and frozen without adding the mozzarella cheese. In the morning, remove from freezer, add cheese, and cook at 350° until cheese is melted.

GRANOLA CEREAL OR BARS

Makes 8 cups

4 cups rolled oats	1 cup chopped nuts
1 cup sesame seeds	½ cup packed brown sugar
1 cup wheat germ	½ cup pure vegetable oil
1 cup shredded coconut	1 cup honey

Oven 250°

Combine all dry ingredients in a large bowl. Mix the oil and honey together and pour over dry ingredients while stirring. Continue to stir until evenly distributed. Spread granola out on two or three cookie sheets and bake in the oven for 30 minutes, stirring about every 10 minutes. Allow the cereal to cool on the baking sheets and then store in airtight containers. The granola will not be crunchy when you take it from the oven but will be after it cools.

To make the mixture into bars, press into the bottom of baking pans until about ⅜ inch deep. Bake in the oven for 30 minutes. As soon as you remove the granola from the oven, cut into bars of desired size with a sharp knife. Allow to cool in the pans. Remove and store bars in airtight containers.

QUICKIE BREAKFAST

Serves 1

1 cup milk
1 banana, sliced
1 raw egg
¼ cup sugar

1 tablespoon wheat germ
(optional)
1 tablespoon cocoa or
carob powder

Put all ingredients except cocoa into a blender and mix. Add cocoa while continuing to mix and blend until smooth.

GOETTA

Serves 12 to 18

1 pound freshly ground
pork
4 cups water
1½ teaspoons salt
¼ teaspoon pepper

3 bay leaves
1 medium onion, finely
chopped
2 cups pinhead oatmeal

Crumble pork into a saucepan and cover with water. Add salt, pepper, bay leaves, and onion and bring to boil. Mash the pork so it is very fine. Add oatmeal and continue to cook over low heat, about 35 minutes. Stir frequently and add more water if necessary. Mixture should be very thick. Pour into a 9×5×3-inch loaf pan. Refrigerate overnight. Cut into ½-inch slices, as needed, and fry until lightly browned and heated through. Serve as a breakfast meat.

HOMEMADE PORK SAUSAGE

Makes 12 patties

2 pounds coarsely ground
  pork shoulder
4 teaspoons sage
½ teaspoon thyme
½ teaspoon marjoram

½ teaspoon dried sweet
  basil
1½ teaspoons salt
½ teaspoon black pepper
⅔ cup water

Combine all ingredients in a large mixing bowl. Mix thoroughly. Shape into twelve patties and fry or place on a cookie sheet and freeze until firm. Package for freezing and use patties as needed.

To cook, place frozen patty in a skillet and fry slowly until fully cooked and slightly browned.

BREAKFAST CASSEROLE

Serves 6

4 slices bread, cubed
½ pound Homemade Pork
  Sausage* (4 patties)
1 cup grated sharp
  uncolored cheese

6 eggs
1 cup milk
½ teaspoon dry mustard
½ teaspoon salt

Oven 350°

Place the cubed bread in the bottom of a 1½-quart greased casserole dish. Brown the sausage in a skillet and break into small pieces. Drain and sprinkle over the bread cubes. Sprinkle cheese evenly over top. Beat the eggs, milk, mustard, and salt together and pour over the casserole. May be covered and refrigerated overnight. In the morning bake uncovered for 40 to 45 minutes.

ALL-PURPOSE DRY INGREDIENTS MIX

Makes 10 cups

10 cups sifted unbleached flour
5 tablespoons baking powder
5 teaspoons salt

Combine all ingredients together thoroughly and store for future use.

BISCUITS

Makes 12 small or
18 large biscuits

2 cups All-purpose Dry Ingredients Mix*
¼ cup pure vegetable oil
¾ cup milk

Oven 450°

Mix ingredients thoroughly. Turn out on waxed paper and roll out to ½ inch thick. Cut with floured cutter and place close together on greased baking sheet or 1 inch apart for crusty biscuits. Bake for 10 to 12 minutes.

MUFFINS

Makes 1 dozen muffins

2 cups All-purpose Dry
Ingredients Mix*
½ cup pure vegetable oil

1 egg, beaten
¼ cup sugar
¾ cup milk

Oven 400°

Mix ingredients together thoroughly. Mixture will be lumpy. Fill greased muffin cups about two-thirds full. Bake for 25 minutes.

PINEAPPLE OR BLUEBERRY MUFFINS

Makes 1 dozen muffins

Muffins*
½ cup drained blueberries or drained crushed pineapple

Mix batter as for muffins and carefully fold in drained fruit. Bake as for muffins.

PANCAKES

Serves 4

2 cups All-purpose Dry   2 cups milk
   Ingredients Mix*   1 egg
⅓ cup pure vegetable oil

Mix ingredients together thoroughly. Drop by teaspoonfuls onto hot, lightly greased skillet. For thicker pancakes use only 1½ to 1¾ cups milk.

WAFFLES

Makes 4 waffles

2 cups All-purpose Dry   vegetable oil
   Ingredients Mix*   1 egg
3 tablespoons pure   1¾ cups milk

Mix ingredients together thoroughly. Bake on preheated waffle iron until golden brown.

CORN MUFFINS OR CORN BREAD

Makes 1 dozen muffins
or 1 8×8-inch-square
corn bread

1 cup corn meal
1 cup sifted unbleached
  flour
⅓ cup sugar
4 teaspoons baking powder
½ teaspoon salt

1 egg
1 cup milk
¼ cup pure vegetable oil
  or uncolored butter,
  melted

Oven 425°

Sift together all dry ingredients. Add egg, milk, and shortening.
Beat with electric mixer until smooth.

Fill greased muffin cups two-thirds full. Bake 15 to 20 minutes.
Or pour batter into greased 8-inch-square cake pan and bake for
20 to 25 minutes.

CARAMEL SWEET ROLLS

Makes 20 to 24 rolls

1 cup milk
¼ cup uncolored butter,
  melted
5 tablespoons sugar
1 teaspoon salt
1 package dry yeast or 1
  cake compressed yeast

¼ cup warm water
1 egg, beaten (optional)
4 cups unsifted unbleached
  flour
½ cup brown sugar
¼ cup uncolored butter
Finely chopped nuts

Oven 375°

Heat together milk, butter, sugar, and salt until butter is melted.
Cool to lukewarm. In the meantime, dissolve yeast in warm water.
Add dissolved yeast and egg to milk mixture. Add about half the
flour and beat for several minutes with an electric mixer. Work in
remaining flour with spoon. Place in greased bowl, turning dough
to coat the top. Let rise in a warm place until double in bulk,

about 1½ hours. Punch down. With floured hands shape into balls about 1½ inches in diameter.

Place about ½ teaspoon butter and 1 teaspoon brown sugar in each cup of greased muffin pans or paper cupcake holders. A few finely chopped nuts may also be added. Place balls of dough on top, filling cups half full. Let rise until almost double in bulk, about 30 to 45 minutes. Bake for about 12 minutes or until lightly browned on top.

May be frozen wrapped tightly in foil. Defrost. In the morning reheat in foil and serve hot.

SUGAR TOP COFFEE CAKE

Serves 9

¾ cup sugar
¼ cup uncolored butter, softened
1 egg
1 cup milk
1 teaspoon pure vanilla extract
1¾ cups sifted unbleached flour

1 tablespoon baking powder
½ teaspoon salt
1½ cups fresh or frozen (thawed) blueberries, drained (optional)

Topping

½ cup sugar
¼ cup unbleached flour
1½ teaspoons cinnamon
3 tablespoons uncolored butter, melted

½ cup chopped nuts (optional)

Oven 350°

In a bowl mix sugar, butter, and egg thoroughly. Stir in milk and vanilla. Sift dry ingredients together and add to batter. Gently fold in blueberries.

Combine topping ingredients and mix well. Pour batter into a greased 9×9-inch pan and sprinkle with the topping mixture. Bake 40 to 45 minutes. Serve warm. May be reheated or is good cold.

For the lunch box, wrap piece of cake in waxed paper or plastic wrap. Include plastic spoon or fork.

BASIC SWEET YEAST DOUGH

Makes enough dough for
2 large or 3 small cakes

½ cup warm water
2 packages dry yeast or 2
  cakes compressed yeast
1¾ cups scalded milk,
  cooled to lukewarm
½ cup sugar

2 teaspoons salt
½ cup uncolored butter,
  softened
2 eggs
7½ to 8 cups sifted
  unbleached flour

Pour water into a large mixing bowl. Sprinkle yeast on top and mix until dissolved. Add scalded milk, sugar, salt, butter, and eggs. Stir in one half of the flour and mix until smooth. Add enough of the remaining flour so that the dough leaves the sides of the bowl. Knead on a floured board until the dough is very smooth. Put into a greased bowl. Turn the greased side up and cover. Let rise in a warm place until double in bulk, about 1½ hours. Punch down. Divide dough and make into desired shapes. Allow to rise again before baking, as directed in recipes calling for Basic Sweet Yeast Dough.*

CARAMEL NUT COFFEE CAKE

Makes 1 8- or 9-inch cake

½ cup uncolored butter
½ cup packed brown sugar
2 tablespoons light corn
  syrup

½ cup pecan halves
½ recipe Basic Sweet
  Yeast Dough*

Oven 350°

Melt ¼ cup butter in an 8- or 9-inch cake pan. Add the brown sugar, corn syrup, and pecan halves. Stir until combined and the nuts are evenly distributed. Cut the dough into walnut-sized pieces with scissors. Melt the other ¼ cup butter in a small pan. Roll each piece of dough in the butter and place on top of the caramel nut mixture. Place the pieces of dough so they are almost touching. Cover and let rise until almost double in bulk, about 45 minutes. Bake for 30 minutes. Turn the cake over onto a plate when removed from the oven and let stand for a minute to let the topping run down over the rolls. Serve warm.

CINNAMON BUBBLE NUT COFFEE CAKE

Serves 8 to 10

½ cup sugar
1 teaspoon cinnamon
½ recipe Basic Sweet
   Yeast Dough*

½ cup uncolored butter,
   melted
¾ cup finely chopped nuts

Oven 350°

Combine the sugar and cinnamon in a small bowl. Cut the dough into walnut-sized pieces with scissors. Roll each ball in the melted butter, then in the sugar and cinnamon, and finally in the chopped nuts. Place the balls in a greased 10-inch tube pan. Continue with the remainder of the dough making two full layers in the pan. Cover and let rise until almost double in bulk, about 45 minutes. Bake for 30 to 35 minutes. As soon as the cake is removed from the oven, invert onto a plate and remove pan. Break cake into pieces with a fork when ready to serve.

TEA RING

Makes 1 12-inch cake

½ recipe Basic Sweet
   Yeast Dough*
¼ cup uncolored butter,
   softened
½ cup sugar

2 teaspoons cinnamon
1 cup finely chopped nuts
1 cup finely chopped dates
   (optional)

Oven 350°

Roll dough into a 10×20-inch rectangle. Spread evenly with softened butter. Combine sugar and cinnamon together and sprinkle over dough, adding the nuts and dates on top. Roll the dough tightly, starting from the wide side, and pinching the edges to seal. Stretch the dough slightly and place in a ring on a lightly greased baking sheet with seam down. Pinch ends together and cut at 1-inch intervals around the outside of the ring almost through to center. Turn each slice slightly on its side. Cover and let rise until almost double in bulk, about 45 minutes. Bake for 25 to 30 minutes.

5

Packing the Lunch Box

If your child has been buying his lunch at school, he will now have to carry a lunch box or "brown bag it" most days. Younger children seem to enjoy carrying a lunch box filled with a variety of goodies and may be delighted to do so all through grade school. Most older children are happier with a sandwich, a piece of fruit, dessert, or whatever.

However, if you do have prior access to the school menus, you *may* be able to select a rare day now and then when the school lunch should be okay. If you know other parents whose children are on the diet, you might band together to encourage the schools to furnish more foods at least without artificial colorings and flavorings.

Here are some tips for packing your child's lunch to make his meal as delicious and pleasant as possible. Pick the ones appropriate for your child and his personality.

Lunch Box Tips

—Include whatever plastic utensils are needed for his lunch. Holiday or special napkins may cheer his day.
—Include some small surprise on occasion like a yo-yo, small toy, marbles, etc.
—Slip in a small note wishing him a good day and sending your love. Or include an appropriate drawing he'll recognize.
—Buy an inexpensive joke book and each day slip in several jokes he can share with his friends.

—Include miniature salt and pepper shakers. The cardboard ones are prefilled; the plastic ones have to be filled from time to time.

—If you are including a special treat like taffy, send enough pieces so he can share with his friends.

Food Tips

—If your child is "brown bagging it," have him buy his white milk at school. A small disposable container of chocolate or carob syrup may be included so he can make his own chocolate milk.

—Vary his lunch from day to day unless he particularly enjoys the same food over and over.

—Try to pack only those foods he really likes.

—Prepare as much of the lunch box as possible the night before to save yourself time in the morning. Sandwich spreads may be made and stored. Sliced meat sandwiches may be made up in quantity and frozen. They'll keep well up to one month. Label each. Place one in the lunch box in the morning and it will be defrosted by noon. Freezing egg salad or similar sandwiches doesn't work out well.

—Pack lettuce leaves separately from the sandwich so they can be added just before eating. Otherwise they'll wilt and be unappetizing.

—Hot dishes like chili, stew, macaroni and cheese may be packed in a wide-mouth thermos. Include "safe" crackers as desired and necessary utensils.

—Likewise, cold foods like mock applesauce, puddings, cottage cheese, milk shakes, and gelatin desserts may also be packed in a wide-mouth thermos.

—Pack your child's favorite soups in a thermos. Include crackers and spoon.

—For variety, pack a half sandwich with one filling and a half sandwich with another filling. Or make one half sandwich with one kind of bread and use another bread for the other half.

—Spread sandwich filling between buns for variety.

—Several thin slices of meat in a sandwich taste much better than one thick slice and make the sandwich easier to eat.

—Butter bread before spreading with salads made with mayonnaise to prevent soggy sandwiches.

—Instead of always packing sandwiches, some days pack a piece of meat (like fried chicken). Include a special bread like pumpkin or cranberry. These breads freeze well. Freeze individually wrapped slices and use as needed. If your child likes cheese, pack cheese and crackers on occasion.

—Bananas are easy to carry and peel. Fresh pears can be packed and eaten with no preparation. The other fruits on the diet are best sent prepared in small containers.

—Include some treats occasionally like additive-free potato chips, corn chips, or pretzels. Check the labels on your local brands. Also peanuts and other nuts may be included if they are additive-free. A small bag of homemade popcorn would also be a treat.

—Carrot sticks and celery sticks add color, variety, and nutrition. A small package of peanut butter may be included. The carrot sticks or the celery may be sent already spread with peanut butter or cream cheese.

—Small cans of fruit juice are easy to send. Include opener. Milk shakes, chocolate milk, malts may make milk more appetizing for your child and increase his daily milk intake if needed.

—Include some "safe" pickles, if desired.

—A hard-boiled egg (salt shaker included) will add nutrition, protein, and iron in particular, to the lunch. Decorate them with felt-tip pens for a chuckle at lunch time.

—For the younger child, cut the sandwiches with cookie cutters or into distinctive shapes for variety.

—Spread thin slices of date-nut bread with cream cheese for a different taste.

Reminder

In preparing the lunch box here is a *partial* list of foods to be avoided, unless using specific safe brands listed in Appendix B.

Luncheon meats
Chocolate milk purchased at school

Most commercial breads, pastries, crackers, etc.
Commercial ice cream, candy
Tomatoes and tomato-containing foods
Cucumbers and cucumber pickles and relish
Commercial mayonnaise, mustard, and colored butter
Commercial pudding, gelatin mixes
Salicylate fruits

CHICKEN NOODLE SOUP

Serves 6

1 3-pound chicken, cut up
6 cups water
2 teaspoons salt
Pepper to taste
1 bay leaf

2 stalks celery, cut up
6 carrots, cut up
1 large onion, minced
1 cup uncooked noodles

Place chicken in a large saucepan. Cover with water and add salt, pepper, and bay leaf. Cover, bring to a boil, and simmer for 1 hour or until chicken is tender. When chicken is done remove from stock. Refrigerate overnight and skim fat from the top of the broth. Reheat broth, add the vegetables, and cook for 35 minutes or until vegetables are almost tender. Skin and bone chicken and cut meat into small pieces. Add chicken and noodles to broth and cook for an additional 15 minutes.

CREAM SOUP

Makes 1½ quarts

¼ cup pure vegetable oil
3 tablespoons unbleached
   flour
2 cups milk
2 cups Chicken Stock* or
   broth

Dash of salt and paprika
2 cups leftover vegetables
   and/or meat chunks

In a heavy saucepan mix cooking oil and flour over low heat. Gradually add milk, stirring constantly. When mixture begins to boil add chicken stock and continue to stir until well mixed and hot. Add seasonings.

Any cooked vegetables may be used. Drain liquid from vegetables and purée in blender or food mill. Add to soup and cook until hot.

CREAM OF GREEN PEA SOUP

Makes 5 cups

1½ 10-ounce packages frozen peas
⅛ teaspoon crushed dried sweet basil
⅛ teaspoon crushed rosemary
⅛ teaspoon crushed savory

1 tablespoon onion powder
4 tablespoons uncolored butter
3 tablespoons unbleached flour
3 cups milk
½ teaspoon salt

Cook peas according to package directions. Purée with herbs and onion powder in blender until smooth or run peas through a food mill.

Make a white sauce by melting butter, stirring in flour, and adding milk gradually. Stir constantly over medium heat until mixture boils and thickens. Add salt. Gradually blend white sauce into pea purée. Reheat to boiling point.

ONION AND POTATO SOUP

Serves 8

¼ cup pure vegetable oil
2 to 3 medium onions, thinly sliced
¾ teaspoon salt
2 tablespoons pure vegetable oil

2 tablespoons unbleached flour
3½ cups milk
2 cups salted diced cooked potatoes
Paprika (optional)

Heat ¼ cup oil in skillet. Add onions and ¼ teaspoon salt. Cook onions until tender, stirring frequently.

In a heavy saucepan mix 2 tablespoons oil and flour. Add 3 cups milk and ½ teaspoon salt. Stir and heat well. Add onions to white sauce. Add potatoes and ½ cup milk. Heat thoroughly. Serve with a dash of paprika on each portion.

TURKEY SOUP

1 turkey carcass, broken up	Salt and pepper to taste
Water	Uncooked rice, noodles, or
Celery, diced	barley, as desired
Carrots, diced	
Fresh or dried onion, chopped	

Place turkey carcass in a Dutch oven or similar large covered pot. Pour water over the bones so that about one half to two thirds of pot is filled. Bring to a boil. Skim. Cover and reduce heat. Simmer for 2 hours. Remove carcass and pick off any bits of remaining meat from the bones. Add meat to stock. Discard carcass. Refrigerate soup overnight. Skim off fat.

Place soup in a heavy pot and add celery, carrots, and onion as desired. Salt and pepper to taste. Bring to a boil. Add rice, barley, or noodles as desired and cook until they are done.

VEGETABLE BEEF SOUP

Makes 1½ quarts

1 beef soup bone	1 cup diced celery
8 cups water	1 cup diced carrots
1 tablespoon salt	1 cup diced potatoes
2 bay leaves	1 cup diced cabbage
¼ teaspoon chili powder	Uncooked rice, barley, or
⅓ cup chopped onion	noodles, as desired

Cook bone with water, salt, and seasonings for 3 hours. Add vegetables. Cover and simmer 1 hour longer. Remove bones and bay leaves. Remove any meat from bones and add to soup. Refrigerate overnight. Skim off fat. Reheat and add rice, barley, or noodles and cook until done.

CHICKEN OR TURKEY SANDWICH SPREAD

Makes 1½ cups

1 cup finely chopped chicken or turkey
1 hard-boiled egg, chopped
⅓ cup chopped celery

2 tablespoons capers or chopped Sweet Zucchini Pickles*
¼ teaspoon salt

Combine all ingredients above and mix well. Spread as desired on buttered bread. Refrigerate any remaining spread in a covered container. If lettuce is desired, pack the leaves separately from the sandwich in the lunch box.

EGG SALAD SANDWICH SPREAD

Makes ½ cup

2 hard-boiled eggs, chopped
1 tablespoon chopped celery
1 tablespoon capers or chopped Sweet Zucchini Pickles*

2 tablespoons Mayonnaise*
¼ teaspoon dry mustard
⅛ teaspoon salt

Mix all ingredients well. Use immediately or refrigerate in a covered container. Spread as desired on buttered bread.

PORK OR VEAL SALAD SPREAD

Makes about 3 cups

2 cups finely chopped
   cooked pork or veal
1 cup diced celery
½ cup chopped stuffed
   olives

¼ teaspoon garlic salt
1 cup Mayonnaise*
½ teaspoon salt
Pepper to taste

Mix all ingredients together and store in refrigerator. When ready to serve, spread on buttered bread.

CREAM CHEESE AND PINEAPPLE SPREAD

Makes about ½ cup

1 3-ounce package cream cheese, softened
2 tablespoons drained canned crushed pineapple

Mix cheese and pineapple together. Use as sandwich filling on Date and Nut Bread* or buttered White Bread.* Refrigerate leftover spread.

SALMON SALAD SPREAD

Makes 3 cups

2 cups drained canned
   salmon
¼ cup diced onion
1 cup diced celery

1 cup Mayonnaise*
½ teaspoon salt
Pepper to taste

Mix all ingredients together and store in refrigerator. Spread on buttered bread when ready to serve.

TUNA SALAD SANDWICH SPREAD

Makes 1 cup

1 7-ounce can tuna,
  drained, flaked
3 tablespoons capers or
  chopped Sweet Zucchini
  Pickles*

2 tablespoons finely
  chopped celery
Mayonnaise*

Mix tuna, pickles or capers, and celery together. Add enough mayonnaise for a moist filling. Quantity of mayonnaise required will depend on whether the tuna is packed in water or oil. Spread on buttered bread when ready to serve. Refrigerate any leftover spread in a covered container.

CHEESE SANDWICH SPREAD

Makes about 2 cups

2 tablespoons uncolored
  butter
2 tablespoons unbleached
  flour
1 cup milk

½ pound uncolored
  cheese, grated
1 egg, slightly beaten
Salt and pepper to taste

Melt butter in a medium saucepan. Remove from heat and blend in the flour. Return to heat and slowly add milk, stirring until smooth and slightly thickened. Add the grated cheese and continue to stir until completely melted. Stir in egg, salt, and pepper. Remove from heat and cool. When cold, spread on slices of bread or crackers. Store leftovers in refrigerator.

This can be prepared and then reheated in the top of a double boiler to serve hot as a cheese sauce to top opened-faced sandwiches.

DEVILED EGGS

Makes 4 half eggs

2 hard-boiled eggs
2 tablespoons
   Mayonnaise*
¼ teaspoon dry mustard
1 tablespoon capers or
   chopped Sweet Zucchini
   Pickles*

Dash of salt
Paprika (optional)

Cut eggs in half. Press egg yolks through sieve. Add mayonnaise, mustard, pickles or capers, and salt. Mix well. Refill eggwhite halves with mixture. Sprinkle with paprika. Refrigerate.

To send eggs in the lunch box, refrigerate until last moment before packing them with the rest of the lunch.

6

Meat, Fish, and Poultry

Preparing your main course at dinner won't present many new problems. Some recipes in this chapter will substitute for prepared items like chicken-coating mixes and stuffing you may have been buying and also for dishes normally prepared with tomatoes. You'll probably have many family favorites too that can be prepared as usual or adapted to the limits of the diet.

Remember to avoid the following:

> Ham or bacon
> Self-basting turkeys
> Prepared breaded frozen fish or chicken
> Purple stamping on meat cuts
> Tomatoes and tomato-based products

Beef

BEEF POT PIE

Serves 4

2 cups cubed leftover pot roast or stew
2 cups leftover gravy, slightly thickened

2 cups leftover peas and/ or carrots (optional)
Salt and pepper to taste
1 recipe Piecrust*

Oven 475°

Combine beef cubes, gravy, vegetables, and seasonings in a round casserole dish. Cover with single pastry crust, pressing dough firmly around the edge of the dish. Prick dough at regular intervals to allow steam to escape. Bake for 15 minutes or until crust is brown around the edge.

BEEF STEW

Serves 6

2 pounds stewing beef, cut up

2 tablespoons pure vegetable oil

Salt to taste

½ cup diced carrots

½ cup diced celery

1 onion, sliced

½ cup 1-inch pieces diced potatoes

½ cup water

¼ cup unbleached flour

Oven 300°

In the bottom of a Dutch oven, brown meat quickly in oil. Barely cover meat with water and salt to taste. Cover and cook in oven for 5 hours. An hour before serving, add carrots, celery, onion, and potatoes. Make a paste of water and flour and add as needed to thicken gravy before serving.

For the lunch box, pour hot stew into a wide-mouth thermos. Include crackers and a plastic spoon or fork in the box.

POT ROAST

Serves 8

1 4-pound blade cut or any other cut suitable for a pot roast

¼ cup unbleached flour seasoned with salt and pepper

2 tablespoons pure vegetable oil

1 cup hot water

8 carrots, cut into chunks

8 peeled potatoes, cut into chunks

1 small onion, sliced

Salt

½ cup water

¼ cup unbleached flour

Oven 300°

Dredge roast in seasoned flour. Brown quickly on all sides in oil. Remove from skillet and place in a Dutch oven or deep casserole. Add hot water and cover tightly. Cook in oven for 4 hours. One hour before serving time add carrots and potatoes. Place slices of onion on meat and salt. When ready to serve, remove meat to platter. Surround with vegetables. Thicken gravy by making a paste of water and flour. Add slowly to gravy, as needed, stirring until it thickens.

SLOW-COOKED ROAST

Slow cooking turns an inexpensive cut of meat into a juicy, tender roast. Allow lots of cooking time. If roast is large, it may be started the night before. You will soon get a feel for the cooking time needed.

1 beef roast, any cut
2 tablespoons uncolored butter or pure vegetable oil

Oven 300°

Early in the day spread meat with butter or coat with oil on all surfaces. Do not season. Place on a rack in a roasting pan. Bake for 1 hour to kill surface bacteria. Reduce heat to about 150° or 160°. Insert a meat thermometer and cook until thermometer registers desired internal temperature indicating degree of doneness. For a beef roast to be medium done, temperature should be about 150°. A five-pound roast, medium done, will require at least 6 hours' total cooking time.

VEAL CUTLETS

Serves 4

1 12-ounce veal cutlet
1 egg
2 tablespoons water

Dry Bread Crumbs*
3 tablespoons pure
   vegetable oil

Oven 325°

Cut cutlet in two. Beat egg and water together. Dip each piece in bread crumbs, then dip in egg mixture. Dip again in crumbs until well coated. Brown cutlets quickly on both sides in oil in a heavy skillet. Cover and bake in skillet for about 50 minutes. Cut into 4 servings.

GOURMET VEAL CUTLETS

Serves 4

Veal Cutlets*
Pesto Sauce*
White cheese

Prepare meat as per veal cutlets recipe. After cutlets are done cooking, spread pesto sauce over cutlets. Top with slices of cheese so that each piece is covered. Broil until cheese is melted and bubbling.

VEAL CHOPS

Serves 4

¼ cup pure vegetable oil
2 medium onions, sliced in thin rings
4 veal chops
Salt and pepper to taste
1 cup Chicken Stock*

1 bay leaf
1 teaspoon dried parsley flakes
¼ cup unbleached flour
½ cup water

Heat oil in heavy skillet or pot. Add sliced onions. Cover and simmer very slowly until transparent, about 15 minutes. Remove onions to side dish. Turn heat up and quickly brown chops on each side. Salt and pepper. Add more oil while browning chops if necessary.

Remove chops and set aside. Pour oil out of skillet. Heat chicken stock in skillet and simmer for 1 minute. Return chops to pan with any juice that collected in dish. Add cooked onions on top of chops and bay leaf and parsley. Cover pan and simmer very slowly for about 30 minutes or until tender. Place chops and onions on a warm platter. Discard bay leaf. Thicken juices in pan with flour mixed with water. Stir until thickened. Pour over chops and onions.

TONGUE

Serves 8 to 10

1 3-pound beef tongue
2 teaspoons salt
3 bay leaves
½ teaspoon nutmeg
½ teaspoon cinnamon
3 whole black peppers

1 tablespoon white distilled
 vinegar
1 onion, sliced
1 carrot, sliced
1 stalk celery, sliced
6 to 8 sprigs fresh parsley

Wash tongue. Cover with boiling water. Add seasonings and vegetables. Simmer uncovered about 3 hours. Cool in cooking liquid. Skin and trim away excess tissue. Slice and serve with Horseradish Sauce.*

For sandwiches, slice thin. Bread may be spread with butter and/or Mayonnaise* and Horseradish Sauce* as desired. Wrap well for lunch box.

Fowl

BARBECUED CHICKEN

Serves 6

2 3-pound chickens, cut up
1 egg
1 cup pure vegetable oil
2 cups white distilled
 vinegar

⅓ cup salt
1 tablespoon poultry
 seasoning
½ teaspoon pepper

Oven 350°

Arrange chicken in a shallow baking dish. Beat the egg and gradually add the oil. Add remaining ingredients and stir thoroughly. Pour marinade over chicken and let stand for at least 1 hour. Drain chicken and either cook on a grill or bake for 1 hour. Baste the pieces of chicken several times while cooking.

BROILED CHICKEN PARTS

Serves 4

4 chicken thighs
4 chicken breasts
⅓ to ½ cup pure vegetable
  oil

2 tablespoons dried parsley ·
  flakes
2 tablespoons frozen or
  dried chopped chives

Line a pan with foil. Place chicken pieces on foil. Combine oil, parsley flakes, and chopped chives. Pour over chicken. Let stand at room temperature for about 1 hour. Drain.

Broil chicken on top rack of oven for 25 to 30 minutes, turning the pieces once.

CHICKEN PIE

Serves 4

2 tablespoons pure
  vegetable oil
¼ cup flour
1 teaspoon salt
Dash of pepper
2 cups Chicken Stock*

2 cups cubed cooked
  chicken
1 cup diced cooked carrots
1 cup cooked peas
1 recipe Piecrust*

Oven 475°

In a large saucepan combine oil and flour over medium heat. Add seasonings and chicken stock. Stir constantly until sauce boils. Turn to simmer and add chicken, carrots, and peas. Pour mixture into a round casserole dish. Place prepared pastry dough on top, pressing edges to sides of casserole dish. At intervals prick crust with a fork to allow steam to escape. Bake 12 to 15 minutes or until crust begins to brown around the edge.

CHICKEN SHAKE

Enough coating for
4 cut-up chickens

4 cups Dry Bread Crumbs*   1 tablespoon salt
½ cup pure vegetable oil   1 teaspoon pepper
1 tablespoon paprika   1 frying chicken, cut up
1 tablespoon celery salt   1 cup water or milk

Oven 375°

Blend crumbs and oil thoroughly in a mixing bowl. Add seasonings and mix well. Store in a covered container in the refrigerator. Use about 1 cup of the mixture for one cut-up frying chicken.

Place mixture in a paper bag. Dip chicken pieces in water or milk. Shake off excess. Shake two to three pieces at a time in the mixture until well coated. Place coated chicken on a cookie sheet. Bake about 50 to 60 minutes. Cover lightly with foil toward end of cooking time if necessary. Serve hot.

Wrap one or more cold chicken pieces for the lunch box. Include a package of salt, if desired.

CHICKEN TURNOVERS

Makes 6 turnovers

Double recipe Piecrust*   ⅛ teaspoon poultry
1 cup finely chopped   seasoning
   cooked chicken   Salt and pepper to taste
½ cup chicken gravy   2 tablespoons milk
¼ cup chopped
   mushrooms

Oven 350 °

Prepare piecrust and divide in two. Roll each half out between sheets of waxed paper and cut the pastry into 5-inch squares.

Combine chicken with rest of the filling ingredients except milk and mix well. Divide chicken mixture evenly onto the pastry squares. Fold pastry over the top of the filling and seal by pressing edges together with a fork. Brush the top of the turnovers with milk and place on a greased cookie sheet. Bake for 20 to 25 minutes or until golden brown. Serve hot or freeze for future use.

For the lunch box, pack the frozen turnover in the morning and by noon it will be thawed for lunch.

FRIED CHICKEN

Serves 4 to 6

1 cup unbleached flour	½ cup pure vegetable oil
2 teaspoons salt	1 2½- to 3-pound frying
1 teaspoon poultry	chicken, cut up
seasoning	¼ cup water
1 cup milk	

Combine in a plastic bag the flour, salt, and poultry seasoning. Dip chicken in milk and shake a few pieces at a time in bag with flour until well coated. Heat oil in skillet and brown chicken on all sides. Reduce heat, add water, cover, and continue to cook chicken about 40 to 45 minutes or until tender. Remove cover and cook an additional 10 minutes until crispy.

Chicken can also be cooked by baking in a 350° oven for 45 minutes after browning in skillet. This gives a very crisp crust.

PINEAPPLE CHICKEN

Serves 6

1 2½- to 3-pound frying	1 cup milk
chicken	½ cup pure vegetable oil
¾ cup unbleached flour	1 cup crushed sweetened
2 teaspoons salt	pineapple with juice
1½ teaspoons ginger	½ cup water

Cut chicken into serving pieces. Combine the flour, salt, and ginger in a bag. Dip chicken pieces in milk and coat with flour mixture. Brown in a skillet with the oil a few pieces at a time. Return all the pieces to the skillet and pour the pineapple mixed with the water over all. Cover and simmer gently for 45 minutes. Uncover and cook an additional 15 minutes or until tender.

STEWED CHICKEN

Serves 6

6 chicken breasts
4 stalks celery, including
  leaves, chopped

4 carrots, sliced
¼ cup instant minced
  onion

Place chicken in a Dutch oven. Add chopped celery, sliced carrots, and onion. Cover with boiling water. Cover the pot and bring to a boil, then turn to simmer. Cook until tender, 1½ hours. Test with a fork for tenderness. Chicken may be served with a little of the stock poured over the pieces.

The stock which is left may be strained to remove vegetables. Store in a covered container in refrigerator. The next day remove hardened fat from the top. Stock may be used in other recipes or served as chicken broth.

TACO CHICKEN

Serves 4 to 6

1½ cups Dry Bread
  Crumbs*
1 1¾-ounce package taco
  mix (additive-free)

1 2½- to 3-pound frying
  chicken, cut up
1 cup evaporated milk

Oven 350°

Mix the bread crumbs and taco mix together in a plastic bag. Dip the pieces of chicken in evaporated milk and put them two at a time in the bag with the taco mixture. Coat the chicken and place on a shallow baking pan. Bake for 1 hour or until tender. Serve hot or send cold leftover chicken pieces wrapped well in the lunch box.

ROAST CHICKEN, CAPON, OR TURKEY IN FOIL

1 chicken, capon, or   1 tablespoon salt
   turkey, at room   Stuffing*
   temperature   Uncolored butter

Oven 400°

Wash bird thoroughly inside and out. Dry well. Rub salt inside
the bird. Fill cavity with stuffing. Tie legs together and wings together. Place on large sheet of heavy-duty foil. Rub legs and
breast with butter. Fold foil to cover bird completely. If necessary
use more foil over breast.

Roast in a large pan for 20 minutes. Reduce heat to 350°. For
a chicken or capon, allow 25 minutes per pound. A turkey under
10 pounds also requires 25 minutes per pound. A larger turkey
needs only 20 minutes per pound. About 30 to 45 minutes before
the bird is done, open and fold back foil. Baste frequently with
pan drippings as bird browns.

ROCK CORNISH HENS

Serves 4

2 tablespoons pure lemon   4 Cornish hens, at room
   juice   temperature
½ cup pure vegetable oil   Salt and pepper to taste

Oven 350°

Mix lemon juice and oil thoroughly. Place hens in roasting pan.
Coat with oil mixture. Bake. After 30 minutes salt and pepper
hens. Baste. Bake 20 minutes longer. Turn oven temperature to
400° and bake 10 more minutes or until done and lightly
browned. Baste with more oil if necessary during cooking.

STUFFING

Enough for 10-pound turkey

1½ teaspoons poultry
    seasoning
¼ teaspoon nutmeg
2 teaspoons salt
8 cups small pieces dried
    bread

2 tablespoons grated onion
2 eggs, slightly beaten
½ cup pure vegetable oil

Combine dry ingredients with bread pieces. Add onion, eggs, and oil. Mix well.

Fish

EASY BAKED FISH

Serves 4

24 ounces any inexpensive
    frozen fish fillets (thawed)
    (cod is delicious this way)
Mayonnaise*
Soft Bread Crumbs*
    seasoned with salt and
    pepper

Salt
Paprika
Dried parsley flakes

Oven 500°

Spread fish fillets with mayonnaise. Roll in seasoned soft bread crumbs. Place in a well-greased pan. Sprinkle each fillet with salt, paprika, and parsley. Bake for 10 minutes. Test with fork to be sure fish flakes easily and is done. Serve with lemon wedges or Tartar Sauce.*

FISH CHOWDER

Makes 2 quarts

1 cup finely diced carrots
1 cup diced uncooked
   potatoes
1 cup chopped onion
½ cup finely diced celery
1 bay leaf
1½ cups water
1 12-ounce package frozen
   fish fillets (thawed)

¼ cup pure vegetable oil
¼ cup unsifted unbleached
   flour
2 teaspoons salt
3½ cups milk
Dried parsley flakes

In a large saucepan place carrots, potatoes, onion, celery, and bay leaf. Add water and bring to a boil. Turn to simmer and cook 15 minutes. Add fish and cook 15 minutes longer. With a fork break fish into small chunks. Discard bay leaf. Cover pan and set aside.

Heat oil in another saucepan, add flour, salt, and mix. Stir in milk gradually. Cook over medium heat, stirring constantly until mixture bubbles. Combine with fish mixture. Serve hot with sprinkling of parsley flakes.

This is a delicious soup or it may be served as a main course for supper.

PLAIN BAKED FISH

Oven 350°

Line a shallow pan with aluminum foil. Place fillets in pan, brush with a little oil, and sprinkle well with paprika. Bake for about 15 minutes for thin fillets, 20 minutes for thicker ones. Test with a fork to be sure fish flakes easily and is done.

TUNA AND CHEESE PIE

Serves 4 to 6

1 recipe Piecrust*
1 6½-ounce can tuna fish, drained
6 ounces grated white cheese
2 tablespoons instant minced onion
2 eggs, beaten

1 cup evaporated milk
1 tablespoon pure lemon juice
1 teaspoon dried chives
1 clove garlic, peeled and minced
1 teaspoon salt
⅛ teaspoon pepper

Oven 450°

Prepare piecrust. Bake for 5 minutes. Sprinkle tuna, cheese, and onion over crust. Combine eggs, milk, lemon juice, and seasonings. Pour over tuna. Bake 15 minutes. Reduce oven to 350° and continue baking another 12 to 15 minutes or until top is lightly browned.

SALMON LOAF

Serves 4

1 16-ounce can salmon
½ cup chopped onion
¼ cup pure vegetable oil
⅓ cup salmon liquid
⅓ cup Dry Bread Crumbs*

2 eggs, beaten
¼ cup chopped parsley
1 teaspoon dry mustard
½ teaspoon salt

Oven 350°

Drain salmon and save liquid. Flake salmon. Add other ingredients and mix well. Place in greased 9×5×3-inch loaf pan. Bake 40 to 50 minutes or until firm in the center. Remove from oven and let stand 5 minutes for easier slicing. Garnish with lemon wedges.

For sandwiches, slice cold salmon loaf into thin slices. Spread bread with butter and/or Mayonnaise.* Wrap well for lunch box.

Ground Meats

CHICKEN PATTIES

Serves 4

¼ cup uncolored butter
¼ cup unbleached flour
1 cup milk
3 cups ground cooked
   chicken
1 tablespoon minced
   parsley
1 teaspoon salt

¼ teaspoon pepper
1 tablespoon grated onion
1 egg, slightly beaten
2 teaspoons water
1 cup Dry Bread Crumbs*
½ cup pure vegetable oil
1 cup chicken gravy

Melt butter in a medium saucepan. Stir in flour. When mixture is smooth, slowly add milk and continue to stir until sauce is thickened. Remove from heat and add ground chicken, parsley, salt, pepper, and onion. Spread mixture around the bottom and sides of pan and refrigerate for several hours until thoroughly chilled. When ready to cook, shape chicken into eight patties. In a shallow dish combine the egg and water. Dip the patties quickly into the egg mixture and then into the dry bread crumbs, pressing crumbs onto the patties until fully covered. Fry in a heavy skillet over medium heat until brown. Serve hot and topped with chicken gravy.

HAMBURGER PIE

Serves 4

1 heaping cup (½ pound)
   sliced cleaned
   mushrooms
2 tablespoons pure
   vegetable oil
¼ cup chopped onion
¼ cup chopped green
   pepper

1 pound ground beef
½ teaspoon salt
Dash of pepper
⅛ teaspoon chili powder
1 recipe Piecrust,* baked
White cheese
Paprika

Oven 350°

Brown mushrooms in a small amount of oil. Set aside. In the same skillet, adding more oil if needed, brown chopped onion and green pepper. Add ground beef, salt, pepper, and chili powder. Simmer for 20 minutes. Using a slotted spoon to drain off oil, place mixture in pie shell. Spread mushrooms on top and over that place slices of white cheese until top is covered. Sprinkle with paprika. Bake for 15 minutes.

ITALIAN HAMBURGERS

Ground lean beef
Pesto Sauce*
White cheese

Form ground beef into patties. Broil on one side. Turn patties over and spread pesto sauce over each one. Return to the broiler. When nearly done place slices of white cheese on top of each. When cheese has melted, remove from oven and serve.

ITALIAN SAUSAGE

Makes 1½ pounds

1½ pounds coarsely
    ground pork
1 teaspoon garlic salt
1 teaspoon fennel seed
½ teaspoon salt
½ teaspoon Italian
    seasoning

½ teaspoon chili powder
⅛ teaspoon pepper
2 tablespoons water
2 tablespoons pure vegetable
    oil

Combine all ingredients, except oil, so spices are evenly distributed. Shape into patties. Fry, using a little oil, until fully cooked.

This is delicious on pizzas. Instead of shaping into patties, crumble sausage into skillet and brown. Sprinkle over pizza sauce and top with mozzarella cheese.

LAYERED MEAT LOAF

Serves 6

Filling

2 cups Soft Bread Crumbs*
½ cup chopped celery
1 tablespoon instant
  minced onion
1 tablespoon pure
  vegetable oil

1 tablespoon minced
  parsley
1 teaspoon salt
¼ teaspoon pepper

1½ pounds ground beef
1½ teaspoons salt
½ teaspoon pepper

1 egg, beaten
½ cup bread crumbs
½ cup milk

Oven 350°

Mix together all the filling ingredients. In another bowl, combine meat loaf ingredients. Spread one half of the meat loaf mixture in a 9×5×3-inch loaf pan. Spread with filling and put the remaining meat mixture on top. Bake for 1 hour.

Serve hot or cold. It is not good for a sandwich filling but may be packed in slices in a lunch box.

MEAT LOAF I

Serves 4

¾ pound ground lean beef
½ cup Dry Bread
  Crumbs*
⅔ cup milk
1 egg, beaten
2 tablespoons chopped
  onion (optional)

⅛ teaspoon pepper
⅛ teaspoon dry mustard
⅛ teaspoon celery salt
⅛ teaspoon garlic salt

Oven 350°

Mix all ingredients. Make into two small loaves. Place in shallow greased pan. Bake 1 hour. Recipe may be doubled to make four loaves to be used for sandwiches.

For sandwiches, slice the cold meat loaf into thin slices. Bread may be spread with uncolored butter and/or Mayonnaise,* Hot Mustard,* or Catsup I* or II.* Wrap well for lunch box.

MEAT LOAF II

Serves 6

1½ pounds ground beef
¾ cup Dry Bread
   Crumbs*
1 cup milk
1 egg, beaten
1 tablespoon onion powder
¼ teaspoon pepper
1 teaspoon salt

¼ teaspoon dry mustard
¼ teaspoon celery salt
¼ teaspoon garlic salt
¼ teaspoon sage
⅛ teaspoon Tabasco sauce
1 tablespoon uncolored soy
   sauce

Oven 350°

Combine all ingredients and mix thoroughly. Shape into a loaf. Place in a shallow pan and bake 1 to 1½ hours.

Slice cold meat loaf into thin slices for sandwiches. Bread may be spread with butter, and/or Mayonnaise,* Hot Mustard,* or Catsup I* or II.* Wrap well for lunch box.

PESTO OR PARSLEY SPAGHETTI

Serves 4

8 ounces spaghetti
Pesto* or Parsley Sauce*

½ pound ground beef
Grated Parmesan cheese

Cook spaghetti according to package directions. Prepare pesto or parsley sauce. Brown ground beef in a heavy skillet. Drain off any excess grease. Add parsley or pesto sauce and heat through. Pour over cooked spaghetti and serve topped with grated Parmesan cheese.

SWEET AND SOUR MEAT BALLS

Serves 4

1 egg, slightly beaten
¾ pound ground beef
¼ cup milk
½ cup Soft Bread
    Crumbs*
1½ teaspoons instant
    minced onion

½ teaspoon salt
⅛ teaspoon pepper
¼ cup packed brown sugar
½ teaspoon dry mustard
½ cup water
¼ cup white distilled
    vinegar

Oven 325°

In a large mixing bowl combine egg, ground beef, milk, bread crumbs, onion, salt, and pepper. Mix well and shape into balls, using about 1 tablespoon of mixture for each ball. Place side by side in a greased baking dish. In a small saucepan, combine brown sugar, dry mustard, water, and vinegar. Place on medium heat and stir until mixture is hot and sugar dissolved. Pour over meat balls. Bake uncovered for 1 hour. Baste with sauce every 15 minutes.

TOMATO-LESS CHILI

Serves 4 to 6

½ pound dried kidney
    beans
1 large onion, chopped
1 green pepper, chopped
1 pound ground beef
1½ tablespoons chili
    powder

1½ teaspoons salt
¼ teaspoon pepper
1 bay leaf
⅛ teaspoon paprika
½ cup water
¼ cup unbleached flour

Prepare dried kidney beans according to directions on package. In a deep skillet brown onion, green pepper, and beef. Add cooked beans, including the liquid in which they were cooked. Add chili powder, salt, pepper, bay leaf, and paprika. Simmer covered 1½ hours. Just before serving, make a paste of water and flour and add to chili if it is too thin. Good with grated Parmesan cheese sprinkled on top.

For the lunch box, pour hot chili into a wide-mouth thermos. Include crackers and a plastic spoon in the box.

May also be frozen for future use.

TOMATO-LESS LASAGNE

Serves 4 to 6

8 ounces uncooked lasagne
  noodles
¾ pound lean ground beef
¾ cup Pesto Sauce*
1 teaspoon Italian
  seasoning

¼ cup minced onion
1½ cups cottage cheese
8 ounces mozzarella
  cheese, shredded
¼ cup grated Parmesan
  cheese

Oven 350°

Prepare lasagne noodles according to package directions. In the meantime, brown beef and add pesto sauce, Italian seasoning, and onion. Bring to a boil and simmer for 10 minutes.

In a greased 8×8-inch baking dish, place one layer of noodles. Add half the meat mixture and half the cottage cheese. Add another layer of noodles. Place half the mozzarella cheese, remaining meat, and remaining cottage cheese in layers. Add the last noodles and cover with mozzarella cheese. Sprinkle with Parmesan cheese. Bake for 20 to 25 minutes or until the cheese is just melted.

Lamb

BROILED LAMB CHOPS

Serves 4

4 rib lamb chops
Salt and pepper to taste
Garlic powder

Sprinkle both sides of rib lamb chops with salt, pepper, and garlic powder. Slash fat edge at 1-inch intervals. Place on rack in broiler pan so chops are 3 inches from preheated broiler. Broil 5 to 7 minutes on each side.

LAMB STEW

Serves 6

2 pounds lamb, cubed
¼ cup unbleached flour
  seasoned with salt and
  pepper
4 to 6 tablespoons pure
  vegetable oil

½ cup sliced onions
1 cup sliced carrots
1 cup diced celery
½ cup water
¼ cup unbleached flour

Coat lamb cubes with seasoned flour. In a heavy saucepan brown them quickly in oil. Drain cubes on paper towels. Brown onions in remaining oil over medium heat. Return lamb to the pot and cover with boiling water. Cover the pot and simmer for about 2 hours. Add carrots and celery. Bring to a boil, then simmer for ½ hour. Thicken stock with a mixture of water and flour, stirred in slowly. Salt and pepper to taste. Good served over hot rice.

Pork

BUTTERFLY PORK CHOPS

Serves 4

4 butterfly pork chops or 4 loin or shoulder pork chops
¼ cup unbleached flour seasoned with salt and pepper
3 tablespoons pure vegetable oil

Oven 275°

Dip chops in seasoned flour. In a heavy skillet over medium heat brown chops in oil for about 10 minutes. Cover and cook in oven for 50 minutes more. Turn every 10 minutes.

PORK CHOPS, SWEET AND SOUR

Serves 6

6 pork chops
1 teaspoon ginger
1 teaspoon salt
½ teaspoon pepper
½ teaspoon paprika
¼ cup unbleached flour

3 tablespoons pure
vegetable oil
1 cup pineapple juice
2 tablespoons white
distilled vinegar
3 tablespoons brown sugar

Oven 275°

Coat both sides of chops with mixture of ginger, salt, pepper, paprika, and flour. In a skillet brown chops in oil over low heat, turning once. Mix together other ingredients and pour over chops. Cover skillet. Place in oven and cook chops 1 hour or until tender. A covered baking dish may be used instead of the skillet for the oven baking.

STUFFED PORK CHOPS

Serves 4

4 pork chops, cut 1 inch
thick
1 cup Stuffing*

¼ cup pure vegetable oil
¾ cup milk
Salt and pepper to taste

Oven 350°

Cut pockets in the pork chops and stuff, using toothpicks to hold edges together. In a heavy skillet brown chops on both sides in oil. Place chops in an ovenproof dish, pour milk, salt, and pepper over all, and bake, covered, for 1 hour or until tender.

SPARERIBS WITH CRANBERRY MARINADE

Serves 4

1½ cups cranberry juice
   cocktail
½ cup packed brown sugar
1 medium onion, thinly
   sliced
1 tablespoon pure lemon
   juice

1 teaspoon salt
⅛ teaspoon pepper
¼ teaspoon ginger
½ teaspoon uncolored soy
   sauce
4 pounds lean spareribs

Oven 350°

Combine all ingredients except spareribs in a saucepan and simmer slowly for 5 minutes. Place ribs in a shallow dish and pour hot cranberry mixture over them. Marinate in refrigerator for at least 3 hours. When ready to cook, drain off juice, pour ½ cup marinade over spareribs, and cover loosely with foil. Bake for 1½ hours. Every ½ hour pour some of the remaining sauce over the ribs. Uncover for the last 20 to 30 minutes to brown.

7

Casseroles

Your family may or may not enjoy casserole dishes. If they do, you'll no doubt be able to use or adapt some of your family favorites. This chapter may give you some other ideas too.

Remember to avoid the following:

> Tomatoes and tomato-based products
> Bleached white flour
> Purple stamping on meat
> Colored butter or margarine

Fowl

CHICKEN CASSEROLE

Serves 4

2 cups cubed cooked
  chicken
2 cups finely chopped
  celery
1 teaspoon salt
2 tablespoons grated onion
1½ teaspoons pure lemon
  juice

1 cup Mayonnaise*
½ cup Dry Bread
  Crumbs*
⅓ cup grated Parmesan
  cheese

Oven 350°

Mix all ingredients except bread crumbs and cheese. Place in a greased 2-quart casserole. Sprinkle crumbs and cheese over top. Bake for 30 minutes or until heated through and lightly browned.

CHICKEN AND BROCCOLI CASSEROLE

Serves 4

1 10-ounce package frozen broccoli
½ cup mushroom pieces (optional)
3 tablespoons pure vegetable oil
1 cup cubed cooked chicken
1 tablespoon unbleached flour

½ cup milk
Salt and pepper to taste
½ cup sour cream
½ cup Mayonnaise*
½ teaspoon instant minced onion
½ teaspoon pure lemon juice
Buttered Soft Bread Crumbs*

Oven 350°

Cook broccoli according to package instructions. Cook mushrooms in 2 tablespoons oil over medium heat until golden brown. Set aside on a paper towel. In a greased 2-quart casserole, place broccoli. Mix cooked chicken with mushrooms and cover the broccoli. In a saucepan mix 1 tablespoon oil and flour and add milk. Stir constantly over medium heat until sauce boils. Remove from heat. Lightly salt and pepper the sauce, add sour cream, mayonnaise, onion, and lemon juice. Stir until well mixed. Pour over casserole. Spread buttered Soft Bread Crumbs* on top. Bake for 30 minutes.

CHICKEN AND POTATO CASSEROLE

Serves 6

4 cups sliced peeled
potatoes
2 cups cubed cooked
chicken
1 10-ounce package frozen
peas
¼ cup uncolored butter
¼ cup unbleached flour

1 cup Chicken Stock*
1 cup milk
1 tablespoon instant
minced onion
¼ teaspoon dry mustard
2 teaspoons salt
⅛ teaspoon pepper
Dash of Tabasco sauce

Oven 375°

Place a layer of 2 cups sliced potatoes in the bottom of an
11×7×2-inch greased casserole and cover with cubed chicken.
Pour frozen peas over chicken and top with remaining potatoes.

Melt butter in a saucepan and blend in flour. Slowly add
chicken stock and milk and cook until thickened. Add onion,
mustard, salt, pepper, and Tabasco. Pour evenly on top of potatoes. Bake for about 1 hour or until potatoes are done. If the potatoes start to brown too much, cover for the last few minutes
with aluminum foil.

CHICKEN AND RICE CASSEROLE

Serves 6

2 cups cooked rice
½ cup cooked chopped
mushrooms (optional)
2 cups diced cooked
chicken
1 cup finely diced celery
2 tablespoons pure
vegetable oil

2 tablespoons unbleached
flour
1 cup milk
1 tablespoon pure lemon
juice
1 cup sour cream
Salt and pepper to taste
Grated Parmesan cheese

Oven 400°

Mix rice and mushrooms together. In a greased casserole place half the mixture. Combine chicken and celery and place on top. Cover with the rest of rice and mushrooms.

In a saucepan heat oil. Blend with flour and milk over medium heat, stirring constantly until sauce boils. Remove from heat. Add lemon juice and gently stir in sour cream. Pour over casserole. Salt and pepper lightly. Sprinkle with enough Parmesan cheese to cover. Bake for 25 minutes or until lightly browned.

CHICKEN-MACARONI CASSEROLE

Serves 6

3 tablespoons pure
    vegetable oil
3 tablespoons unbleached
    flour
1 cup Chicken Stock* or
    broth
1 cup milk
Salt and pepper to taste

1 cup uncooked macaroni,
    cooked and drained
2 cups diced cooked
    chicken
1 teaspoon frozen or dried
    chopped chives
    (optional)
Grated Parmesan cheese

Oven 375°

In a large saucepan combine oil and flour. Add chicken stock and cook over medium heat, stirring constantly. Gradually pour in milk and continue stirring until mixture boils. Set aside and season with salt and pepper. Stir in cooked macaroni, chicken, and chives. Pour ingredients into a large greased casserole. Top generously with Parmesan cheese. Bake for 30 minutes.

CREAMED CHICKEN

Serves 4

2 tablespoons pure
  vegetable oil
2 tablespoons unbleached
  flour
1 cup milk
½ teaspoon salt

⅛ teaspoon paprika
1 teaspoon frozen or dried
  chopped chives
2 cups diced cooked
  chicken

In a saucepan mix oil and flour. Add milk and bring to a boil, stirring constantly. Add salt, paprika, and chives. Stir in chicken and simmer for a few minutes until chicken is heated. Stir so the sauce does not stick to the pan.

Serve mixture over rice, noodles, or atop buttered toast.

TURKEY CASSEROLE

Serves 8

2 10-ounce packages
  frozen broccoli, cooked
Salt and pepper to taste
2 cups cubed cooked
  turkey
¼ cup pure vegetable oil
¼ cup unbleached flour
2 cups milk
1 teaspoon salt

½ teaspoon instant minced
  onion
1 cup Mayonnaise*
1 teaspoon pure lemon
  juice
½ cup buttered Dry Bread
  Crumbs*
½ cup grated uncolored
  cheese

Oven 325°

Place cooked, well-drained broccoli in greased 2-quart casserole. Season with salt and pepper. Cover with turkey.

In a saucepan mix oil, flour, and milk over medium heat. Stir constantly until mixture boils. Add salt, onion, mayonnaise, and lemon juice. Pour over turkey. Top with buttered crumbs and grated cheese. Bake uncovered for 25 minutes or until lightly browned.

Beef

BEEF AND VEGETABLE CASSEROLE

Serves 4

¼ cup chopped onion
¼ cup chopped green
  pepper
¾ to 1 pound ground beef
¼ cup pure vegetable oil
¼ cup chopped celery
½ teaspoon salt
Pepper to taste

2 cups any leftover
  vegetables (beans, corn,
  peas, etc.)
Stuffed olives, sliced
  (optional)
Uncolored cheese
Paprika

Oven 350°

In a heavy skillet sauté onion, green pepper, and ground beef in oil. Add celery and seasonings and simmer for 15 minutes, stirring occasionally. Add vegetables, more oil if needed, and cook 5 more minutes. With a slotted spoon place mixture in a greased 1½-quart casserole. Place sliced olives on top. Cover with slices of cheese. Sprinkle with paprika. Bake 15 minutes.

CURRIED VEAL CASSEROLE

Serves 4

2½ tablespoons pure
  vegetable oil
2 tablespoons unbleached
  flour
⅓ cup heavy cream
⅔ cup Chicken Stock*
Salt and pepper to taste

1¼ pounds lean veal,
  cubed
½ teaspoon instant minced
  onion
½ cup sour cream
½ teaspoon salt
1 teaspoon curry powder

Oven 325°

Make a cream sauce by stirring 1 tablespoon oil and 1 table-spoon flour together in saucepan over moderate heat. Add cream, stirring continually. Then add ⅓ cup chicken stock. When thick and bubbling, season and set aside.

Brown veal cubes in remaining 1½ tablespoons oil. Remove meat and place in greased casserole. Add remaining 1 tablespoon flour to skillet. Stir until slightly brown, add onion. Pour in cream sauce, sour cream, remaining ⅓ cup chicken stock, salt, and curry powder. Stir until thoroughly mixed. Pour over veal in the casserole. Stir lightly and cover. Bake for 1½ hours. Serve over rice.

SHEPHERD'S PIE

Serves 6

3 to 4 cups cubed cooked
  beef
1 small onion or 1
  tablespoon instant
  minced onion

1½ cups leftover gravy
1 cup cooked vegetables
Salt and pepper to taste
4 cups leftover mashed
  potatoes

Oven 350°

Combine beef, onion, gravy, and vegetables in a saucepan and heat to boiling. Season with salt and pepper. Spread 2 cups mashed potatoes in a greased 1½-quart casserole. Pour beef mixture over potatoes and spoon the remaining 2 cups potatoes on top. Bake in oven for 30 minutes until potatoes are lightly browned.

Fish

FISH CASSEROLE

Serves 4

2 tablespoons pure
  vegetable oil
2 tablespoons unbleached
  flour
1 cup milk
½ teaspoon salt
1½ teaspoons instant
  minced onion

1 cup grated white cheese
1 16-ounce package frozen
  fish fillets, defrosted and
  drained
¾ cup buttered Dry Bread
  Crumbs*

Oven 350°

In a saucepan, mix oil and flour. Stir in milk and cook over medium heat, stirring constantly until sauce boils. Add salt, instant onion, and grated cheese. Stir well and remove from heat.

In a greased casserole place defrosted fish, cut into bite-size pieces. Pour the cream sauce over it. Top with buttered crumbs. Bake in the upper part of oven for 30 minutes or until lightly browned.

SALMON CASSEROLE

Serves 4

⅔ cup sour cream
½ cup Mayonnaise*
1 teaspoon curry powder
  (optional)
1 1-pound can salmon,
  drained and flaked

1 medium zucchini, peeled
  and thinly sliced
1 cup finely chopped celery
¼ cup diced onion
Buttered Dry Bread
  Crumbs*

Oven 350°

Combine sour cream, mayonnaise, and curry powder. Set aside. In a greased 1½-quart casserole combine salmon, zucchini, celery, and onion. Cover with sauce. Sprinkle top with bread crumbs. Bake for 25 to 30 minutes.

SEAFOOD CASSEROLE DELUXE

Serves 6

1 pound frozen fish fillets
  (thawed)
1 cup Medium White
  Sauce*
1 tablespoon instant
  minced onion
1 cup shredded uncolored
  cheese

½ cup sour cream
½ cup diced mushrooms
1 cup frozen peas
  (partially thawed)
1 tablespoon parsley flakes
1 cup Dry Bread Crumbs*

Oven 400°

Put fish fillets in a skillet and cover with water. Simmer until fish is done and flakes easily. Drain and break into bite-size pieces.

Prepare Medium White Sauce. Remove from heat and add onion and grated cheese. Stir until cheese melts and mixture is smooth.

Stir in sour cream, mushrooms, peas, and parsley. Add the fish and pour into a greased 1½-quart casserole. Sprinkle dry bread crumbs on top. Bake for 15 to 20 minutes until bubbly.

SHRIMP AND CORN CASSEROLE

Serves 6

1 12-ounce package frozen
  shelled deveined raw
  shrimp
3 eggs
½ cup milk
½ cup sour cream
1 1-pound can cream-style
  corn
1 cup broken bread pieces

⅓ cup chopped onion
2 tablespoons chopped
  green pepper
½ teaspoon salt
½ teaspoon garlic salt
⅛ teaspoon pepper
1 tablespoon pure
  vegetable oil

Oven 350°

Cook shrimp according to directions on label. Drain thoroughly and cut into small pieces. In a large bowl beat eggs. Stir in milk, sour cream, corn, broken pieces of bread, onion, green pepper, salt, garlic salt, pepper, and oil. Mix thoroughly. Add the shrimp and stir well. Turn into a 1½-quart greased casserole. Bake for 1½ hours or until knife inserted in the middle comes out clean.

SHRIMP ORIENTAL

Serves 4

⅓ cup chopped onion
⅓ cup chopped green
pepper
3 tablespoons pure
vegetable oil
1 cup drained bean sprouts
⅓ cup canned mushroom
pieces

1 8-ounce can water
chestnuts, drained and
sliced
1 4½-ounce can shrimp,
drained
3 eggs
½ cup milk
1 teaspoon salt

Oven 350°

Sauté onion and green pepper in oil until partially cooked. Add bean sprouts, mushrooms, water chestnuts, and shrimp and heat through. Pour this mixture into a 1½-quart casserole dish. Combine eggs, milk, and salt in a small bowl and beat until well mixed. Pour the eggs over the shrimp mixture in the casserole. Put the casserole dish in a pan filled with 1 inch of water and bake for 45 to 50 minutes or until a knife inserted in the mixture comes out clean.

SPAGHETTI WITH CLAM SAUCE

Serves 4

¾ pound spaghetti
½ cup chopped onion
1 clove garlic, minced
¼ cup pure vegetable oil
2 8-ounce cans minced
clams, reserving juice

½ cup dried parsley
1 teaspoon dried sweet
basil

Cook spaghetti according to package instructions. In a medium-sized skillet sauté onion and garlic in oil until tender. Add the minced clams and their juice. Stir in parsley and basil. Heat through. Serve over spaghetti.

TUNA AND ZUCCHINI CASSEROLE

Serves 6

2 7-ounce cans tuna,
   drained and flaked
1½ cups milk
½ cup Mayonnaise*
2 eggs, beaten
1 cup shredded sharp white
   cheese
4 teaspoons pure lemon
   juice
2 cups finely chopped
   zucchini (peel if waxed)

2 tablespoons instant
   minced onion
½ teaspoon salt
Dash of pepper
2 slices bread, broken into
   very small pieces
Grated Parmesan cheese
Uncolored butter

Oven 350°

In a large mixing bowl combine tuna, milk, mayonnaise, eggs, shredded white cheese, lemon juice, zucchini, onion, salt, and pepper. Pour mixture into a greased 2-quart casserole. Sprinkle small pieces of bread and Parmesan cheese on top. Dot with butter. Bake for 40 minutes or until top begins to brown.

TUNA SPAGHETTI

Serves 4

¾ pound uncooked
   spaghetti
1 small onion, chopped
1 ounce dried parsley
½ cup pure vegetable oil
1 9¼-ounce can tuna fish,
   undrained and flaked

1 tablespoon pure lemon
   juice
Salt and pepper to taste
Grated Parmesan cheese

Prepare spaghetti according to directions on package. In a heavy skillet sauté onion and parsley in oil until onion is yellow. Add tuna. Stir in lemon juice, salt, and pepper, and warm over low heat. Pour over hot spaghetti and toss to mix. Serve with Parmesan cheese.

8

Salads and Salad Dressings

You'll probably have to make your own salad dressings, but they're easily prepared. You'll also have to make your own gelatin salads and desserts as all the prepared mixes are artificially colored and flavored and seem to be notorious in setting off hyperactive children.

Avoid the following in preparing your salad dressings and salads:

Any vinegar except white distilled
Tomatoes, tomato-based products
Cucumbers, cucumber pickles
Salicylate fruits such as apples, peaches, plums, oranges, etc.
Prepared gelatin mixes
Lemon and lime rinds, if waxed

Gelatin

CRANBERRY GELATIN

Serves 4

1 envelope unflavored gelatin
1¼ cups cranberry juice cocktail

¾ cup boiling water
¾ cup sugar
1 tablespoon pure lemon juice

Sprinkle gelatin over ¼ cup cranberry juice to soften. Add boiling water and sugar. Stir until partially dissolved. Add remaining cranberry juice and lemon juice. Stir again until completely dissolved. Pour into serving dishes or a 1-quart mold and chill until set.

This gelatin is good for salads or desserts. Add 1½ cups chopped fruits or vegetables when partially set and return to refrigerator until firm.

LEMON OR LIME GELATIN

Serves 4

1 envelope unflavored
   gelatin
½ cup cold water

1 cup sugar
6 lemons or limes,
   squeezed for juice

In a saucepan dissolve gelatin in cold water. Stir over medium heat until liquid is clear. Add sugar and stir until dissolved. Remove from heat. In a 2-cup measuring cup pour lemon or lime juice, adding enough water to make 2 cups liquid. Combine with gelatin mixture. Mix well and pour into serving dishes or a 1-quart mold and chill until set.

PAPAYA GELATIN

Serves 6

For use with commercial papaya concentrate.

1 envelope unflavored
   gelatin
⅔ cup commercial papaya
   concentrate, chilled

1⅓ cups boiling water
⅓ cup sugar (optional)

For use with Homemade Papaya Concentrate*:

1 envelope unflavored gelatin
¼ cup cold water
1¾ cups hot Homemade
   Papaya Concentrate*

⅓ cup sugar (optional)

Soften gelatin in cold liquid. Add to hot liquid and stir until gelatin is dissolved. Add sugar and stir until dissolved. Chill.

When gelatin has thickened fold in 1½ cups chopped fruits or vegetables. Pour into serving dishes or 1-quart mold and return to refrigerator until firm. Makes a delicious, colorful salad or dessert.

PINEAPPLE GELATIN

Serves 4

1 envelope unflavored gelatin
½ cup cold water
¼ cup sugar (optional)

1½ cups pineapple juice
½ cup water

In a saucepan dissolve gelatin in cold water. Stir over medium heat until liquid is clear. Add sugar and stir until dissolved. Remove from heat. Add pineapple juice and water. Pour into serving dishes or a 1-quart mold and chill until set.

PINEAPPLE AND GRAPEFRUIT GELATIN

Serves 6

1 envelope unflavored
  gelatin
¼ cup cold water
½ cup hot pineapple juice
½ cup hot grapefruit juice
¼ cup pure lemon juice
¼ cup sugar

¼ teaspoon salt
1 cup drained canned
  grapefruit sections,
  reserving juice
1 cup drained canned
  pineapple tidbits or
  chunks, reserving juice

Soften gelatin in cold water. Dissolve in hot fruit juices. Add lemon juice, sugar, and salt. Refrigerate. When mixture begins to thicken, fold in grapefruit and pineapple. Chill in a covered container. May be packed in a wide-mouth thermos for the lunch box.

MOLDED TUNA SALAD

Serves 6

2 7-ounce cans tuna,
drained and flaked
1 tablespoon chopped
onion
1 tablespoon chopped
green pepper
½ cup chopped celery

2 tablespoons pure lemon
juice
¾ cup Mayonnaise*
1½ teaspoons unflavored
gelatin
2 tablespoons cold water
Paprika

In a large bowl combine tuna, onion, green pepper, chopped celery, lemon juice, and mayonnaise. Soften gelatin in cold water; dissolve over hot water. Stir liquid gelatin into tuna mixture. Turn into a 2-quart mold. Cover and refrigerate.

Line a platter with lettuce, unmolding tuna in the middle. Sprinkle top with paprika. Fill the center with cottage cheese topped with chopped chives. Or fill the center with cold cooked peas seasoned with chives. Garnish the platter with carrot sticks and wedges of hard-boiled eggs. Serve with hot biscuits or rolls. Makes a great main course for a summer supper.

TUNA SALAD

Serves 6

Use the above ingredients but omit the gelatin and water. Cover and chill. Serve on lettuce.

MOLDED VEGETABLE SALAD

Serves 6

1 envelope unflavored
gelatin
½ cup cold water
¼ cup sugar
½ teaspoon salt
2 to 4 tablespoons white
distilled vinegar
1 tablespoon pure lemon
juice
1 cup Chicken Stock or
water
1½ cups raw vegetables

(Two different
vegetables are attractive.
For example, shredded
cabbage and finely diced
green pepper or shredded
carrots and thawed frozen
peas which have not been
cooked.) Or 1½ cups
cooked vegetables (For
example, sliced or diced
carrots and peas or lima
beans and corn.)

Sprinkle gelatin over cold water in a small saucepan. Place over low heat and stir constantly until gelatin has completely dissolved. Remove from heat. Add sugar, salt, vinegar, lemon juice, stock or water. Pour into bowl or a 2-quart mold and refrigerate until mixture becomes partially thickened. Fold in either 1½ cups raw or cooked vegetables. Refrigerate covered until firm. Individual molds can be used.

RED, WHITE, AND BLUE HOLIDAY SALAD

Serves 15

Blue Layer

1 envelope unflavored
gelatin
1 cup blueberry juice
(reserved from 1
15-ounce can
blueberries)

1 cup pineapple juice
(reserved from 1 can
crushed unsweetened
pineapple)
½ cup drained crushed
pineapple

White Layer

1 envelope unflavored
  gelatin
½ cup cold water
1 cup sugar

1 cup half and half cream
3 tablespoons lemon juice
2 cups cottage cheese

Red Layer

1 envelope unflavored
  gelatin
2 cups cranberry juice
  cocktail

½ cup sugar
½ cup drained crushed
  pineapple

Allow 24 hours for preparing salad. First, prepare blue layer by softening gelatin in cold blueberry and pineapple juices. Heat juices over low heat until gelatin dissolves. Chill. When almost firm, fold in crushed pineapple. Pour into bottom of large mold (3 quart size, at least) or into individual molds. Chill until firm.

In the meantime, start preparing white layer. Soften gelatin in cold water. Dissolve gelatin and sugar in hot cream. Add lemon juice. Place cottage cheese in blender on highest speed until creamy. Combine well with gelatin mixture. Cool. Pour on top of blue layer. Chill until firm.

Meanwhile, prepare the red layer by softening gelatin in cold cranberry juice. Add sugar and stir over low heat until gelatin and sugar dissolve. Chill. When almost firm, fold in pineapple. Pour on top of white layer. Chill until firm.

Fruit

FRUIT CUPS

Combine fruit together in any one of the following combinations:
1. Watermelon, cantaloupe, and honeydew melon balls
2. Papayas, pineapple, and shredded coconut
3. Sliced bananas, pineapple chunks, and grapefruit segments

4. Pears and blueberries

Sprinkle banana slices with lemon juice to prevent discoloration. Combine with other fruits and chill before serving.

Fruit cups can be served as an appetizer, salad, or a refreshing summertime dessert.

MOCK APPLESAUCE

Makes 3 cups

3 cups (6 large) pears,
  peeled and sliced
1 cup water
½ cup sugar

1 tablespoon pure lemon
  juice
½ teaspoon cinnamon

In a heavy saucepan cook pears, water, and sugar until boiling. Continue boiling for about 30 minutes until mixture thickens and pears are tender. Stir frequently. Add lemon juice and cinnamon. Cool. Place in blender and blend until consistency is similar to applesauce. Serve with added sugar on top if desired. Refrigerate leftovers. May be packed in wide-mouth thermos for the lunch box.

The taste of this mock applesauce is remarkably like that of real applesauce.

PINEAPPLE AND CABBAGE SALAD

Serves 4

2 cups shredded cabbage
4 ounces well drained, crushed pineapple
Creamy Slaw Dressing*

Mix cabbage and crushed pineapple. Add creamy slaw dressing sparingly. Toss with a fork. If necessary more dressing may be added according to taste.

PINEAPPLE-CHICKEN SALAD

Serves 4

2 cups cubed cooked
  chicken
½ cup diced celery
½ cup drained diced
  pineapple chunks

Mayonnaise*
Salt and pepper to taste
Paprika

In a large bowl combine chicken, celery, pineapple. Add enough mayonnaise to moisten ingredients. Salt and pepper to taste. Serve with paprika sprinkled on top.

PINEAPPLE RING SALAD

Canned pineapple rings
Cream cheese
French Dressing*

Arrange pineapple rings on lettuce. Top with a small ball of cheese. Serve with French dressing.

Vegetable

BEET SALAD

Serves 4

1 cup whole or sliced beets (not Harvard beets), coarsely
  chopped
2 hard-boiled eggs, coarsely chopped
2 tablespoons Mayonnaise*

Combine beets and eggs with mayonnaise and salt to taste. Serve on lettuce. Do not prepare more than an hour before serving.

CABBAGE SALAD

Serves 4

4 cups (½ head) very
thinly sliced or coarsely
chopped cabbage
1 Spanish onion, very
thinly sliced

½ green pepper, coarsely
chopped
½ cup sugar
½ cup Simple Salad
Dressing*

In a large bowl lightly mix cabbage, onion, and green pepper. Sprinkle sugar on top. Slowly pour salad dressing to cover entire top surface. Cover and let stand at room temperature for 1 hour. Refrigerate for 5 to 6 hours. Toss salad thoroughly before serving.

LAYERED SALAD

Lettuce, broken in pieces
Frozen (thawed) peas,
uncooked
Carrots, shredded
Pineapple chunks, well
drained

Bermuda onion rings, very
thinly sliced
Mayonnaise*
Sugar
Cheesy Croutons*
Grated Parmesan cheese

In a large bowl layer lettuce, peas, carrots, pineapple chunks, and onion rings. Place spoonfuls of mayonnaise on this mixture and sprinkle with sugar. Repeat the layers again, adding mayonnaise sprinkled with sugar until desired amount is made. Cover bowl and refrigerate 2 or 3 hours. Before serving, top with croutons and grated Parmesan cheese. Do not toss.

SUMMER DINNER SALAD

Lettuce, torn into bite-size
 pieces
Chicken, cooked and cubed
White cheese, sliced in thin
 strips
Hard-boiled eggs, sliced
Ripe olives, pitted
 (optional)
Avocado, cut in wedges
 (optional)

Radishes, sliced (optional)
Carrots, sliced (optional)
Green pepper, chopped
 (optional)
Onion, sliced (optional)
Cheesy Croutons*
Creamy Salad Dressing or
 desired salad dressing

In a large bowl place pieces of lettuce, cubed chicken, strips of white cheese, and sliced hard-boiled eggs. Add ripe olives, avocado wedges, radishes, carrots, green pepper, and sliced onion to your taste. Toss gently. Add croutons. Pour salad dressing on top. Toss again until all the salad ingredients are coated with dressing.

RAW VEGETABLES WITH DIPS

Raw vegetables are a change from the usual salads. On a large plate or platter arrange groups of carrot sticks, celery cut in 2- or 3-inch lengths, zucchini washed well, peeled if waxed, and cut in short sticks, and cauliflower cut into small pieces. Serve with a dip. Children enjoy finger foods.

VEGETABLE DIP

Makes 1 cup

½ cup Mayonnaise*
½ cup sour cream
1½ teaspoons dill seed
1½ teaspoons parsley
 flakes

1½ teaspoons instant
 minced onion
½ teaspoon celery salt

Combine all ingredients and mix well. Refrigerate in a covered container. Serve as a dip for vegetables, potato chips, a spread for crackers, or as a delicious creamy salad dressing.

ZIPPY CURRY DIP

Makes 1 cup

1 cup Mayonnaise*
1 teaspoon curry powder
¼ teaspoon dry mustard

½ teaspoon garlic salt
½ teaspoon onion salt
2 drops Tabasco sauce

Combine all ingredients and chill. Serve as a dip with raw vegetables.

Others

COLD POTATO SALAD

Serves 6

1 cup Mayonnaise*
1 teaspoon dry mustard
2 teaspoons pure lemon
    juice
¼ teaspoon celery seed
½ teaspoon onion salt
2½ teaspoons sugar

5 cups cold cooked cubed
    potatoes
3 hard-boiled eggs,
    chopped
½ cup chopped celery
Salt and pepper to taste

Combine first six ingredients and mix thoroughly. Place potatoes, eggs, and celery in a large bowl and pour mayonnaise mixture on top. Toss lightly until dressing is evenly distributed. Adjust seasonings by adding salt and pepper to taste.

MACARONI SALAD

Serves 6

1 cup 1-inch pieces
uncooked macaroni
1 tablespoon pure
vegetable oil
2 cups diced celery
2 tablespoons chopped
fresh or frozen chives

1 teaspoon salt
Pepper to taste
¼ cup Mayonnaise*
Paprika

Cook macaroni according to package directions. Drain. After 5 minutes add oil and toss with a fork to mix. Refrigerate for several hours. Add celery, chives, salt, pepper, and mayonnaise. Mix thoroughly with macaroni. Serve on lettuce with a sprinkling of paprika on each serving.

Dressings

CREAMY SALAD DRESSING

Makes 1¾ cups

1 tablespoon pure lemon
juice
½ cup pure whipping
cream
2 tablespoons white
distilled vinegar

1 tablespoon dried parsley
flakes
1 tablespoon onion salt
1 cup Mayonnaise*

Add lemon juice to cream. Mix thoroughly with other ingredients. Refrigerate.

CREAMY SLAW DRESSING

Makes 1 cup

½ cup sour cream
¾ cup Mayonnaise*
1 tablespoon sugar

Mix together thoroughly. Refrigerate in a covered jar.

FRENCH DRESSING

Makes 1⅓ cups

1 teaspoon sugar
2 teaspoons salt
½ teaspoon pepper
1 teaspoon paprika

⅓ cup white distilled
    vinegar
1 cup pure vegetable oil

Combine all the ingredients in a covered jar. Shake thoroughly. Refrigerate. Shake well before using.

CREAMY FRENCH DRESSING

Makes 2 cups

French Dressing*
⅔ cup half and half cream

Pour French dressing in blender. Turn on low speed. Slowly add cream until dressing is thick and creamy. Refrigerate in a covered container. Stir well before serving.

CREAMY ONION OR CREAMY GARLIC DRESSING

Makes 2 cups

French Dressing*
1 teaspoon onion or garlic salt
⅔ cup half and half cream

Prepare French dressing but reduce salt to 1 teaspoon. Add onion or garlic salt. Pour into blender, turn on low speed, and slowly add cream until dressing is thick and creamy. Refrigerate in a covered container. Stir well before serving.

FRUIT SALAD DRESSING

Makes 2 cups

⅔ cup sugar
1 heaping teaspoon paprika
½ teaspoon dry mustard
¼ teaspoon onion salt

½ teaspoon celery seed
1 cup pure vegetable oil
½ cup white distilled
  vinegar

Mix dry ingredients thoroughly. Stir in oil and vinegar. Beat until well blended. Store in covered jar in refrigerator. Best left for 24 hours before using. This is also good with a tossed salad.

SIMPLE SALAD DRESSING

Makes ⅔ cup

¼ cup white distilled
  vinegar
⅓ cup pure vegetable oil

4 teaspoons sugar
1 teaspoon salt
½ teaspoon dry mustard

Combine ingredients in a jar with a lid. Shake well. Refrigerate. Shake again before using.

SWEET FRENCH DRESSING

Makes 1½ cups

½ cup sugar
1 heaping teaspoon paprika
¼ teaspoon dry mustard
1 cup pure vegetable oil

½ cup white distilled
  vinegar
1 piece raw onion
  (optional)

Mix all ingredients together. Place in covered container and refrigerate. Remove onion after several days.

9

Vegetables

Except for tomatoes and cucumbers, you can choose any vegetables your family likes. Avoid using any skins that appear to be waxed—zucchini, peppers, and so on. Sometimes sweet potatoes may be dyed on the outside, so beware. Don't use prepared potato, rice, or pasta mixes.

Remember to avoid the following:

> Tomatoes
> Cucumbers
> Colored butter or margarine
> Frozen vegetables already prepared in butter

Green

ASPARAGUS AND EGG CASSEROLE

Serves 6

¼ cup pure vegetable oil
¼ cup unbleached flour
1 cup milk
½ cup sour cream
¼ cup Mayonnaise*
1 16-ounce can asparagus
   pieces, drained and ¼
   cup liquid reserved

5 hard-boiled eggs, thinly
   sliced
Buttered Dry Bread
   Crumbs*

Oven 350°

In a large saucepan combine oil and flour, stir in milk, and continue to stir over medium heat until sauce begins to boil. Remove from heat and add sour cream, mayonnaise, liquid from asparagus, and salt. Mix well over low heat. Add asparagus. In a greased 2-quart casserole, place three sliced hard-boiled eggs. Pour half the creamed asparagus over them. Add remaining eggs and creamed asparagus. Top with buttered crumbs. Bake for ½ hour or until crumbs begin to brown.

BROCCOLI CASSEROLE

Serves 4

2 tablespoons pure
   vegetable oil
2 tablespoons unbleached
   flour
1 cup milk
¼ teaspoon salt
¼ teaspoon instant minced
   onion

1 10-ounce package frozen
   broccoli pieces, cooked
   and drained
Buttered Dry Bread
   Crumbs*

Oven 350°

In a saucepan over medium heat blend oil and flour. Add milk and bring to a boil, stirring constantly. Add salt and dried onion. Combine with cooked broccoli. Place in a well-greased 1½-quart casserole and top with buttered crumbs. Bake for 30 minutes.

CREAMED PEAS OR CARROTS

Serves 4 to 6

1 tablespoon pure
  vegetable oil
1 tablespoon unbleached
  flour
1 cup milk
¼ teaspoon salt

Dash of pepper
½ teaspoon dried minced
  onion
2 cups drained cooked peas
  or carrots

In a saucepan over medium heat mix oil and flour. Stir in milk and continue stirring until mixture comes to a boil. Add salt, pepper, and onion and cook a minute longer. Stir until well blended. Reduce heat to simmer and add peas or carrots. Cover and allow peas or carrots to heat. Serve in individual sauce dishes.

GREEN BEANS WITH PESTO AND CHEESE

Serves 4

1 12-ounce can cut green beans
1 tablespoon Pesto Sauce*
½ cup grated white cheese

In a saucepan heat the green beans. If necessary add a little water to keep them from sticking. When they reach the boiling point drain off all liquid. (Instead of discarding the liquid, which is full of vitamins, add it to your homemade soup.) Stir in pesto sauce and mix well. Add grated cheese. Cover saucepan and set aside on stove until cheese has melted. Stir ingredients well and serve at once.

LIMA BEANS WITH MUSHROOMS

Serves 4

1 10-ounce package frozen
  lima beans
1 pound mushrooms
½ medium onion, chopped

2 to 3 tablespoons pure
  vegetable oil
Salt and pepper to taste

Cook lima beans as directed on the package. Wipe mushrooms with a damp cloth and slice. Sauté onion in oil, add mushrooms and cook until tender. Drain lima beans (saving vitamin-filled liquid for homemade soups). Add onion and mushrooms. Stir together and salt and pepper to taste.

SPINACH AND RICE

Serves 4 to 6

1 10-ounce package frozen
  chopped spinach
1 cup grated white cheese
1 cup cooked rice
2 tablespoons chopped
  onion

2 tablespoons uncolored
  butter, softened
1 teaspoon salt
Dash of pepper
1 cup milk
2 eggs, beaten

Oven 350°

Cook spinach according to package instructions. Drain. Combine with remaining ingredients. Pour into a 2-quart casserole. Bake for 1 hour.

SPINACH SUPREME

2 10-ounce packages
  frozen chopped spinach
1 cup sour cream or yogurt
1½ teaspoons curry
  powder

⅛ teaspoon thyme
Salt and pepper to taste

Oven 350°

Cook spinach according to package instructions. Drain (reserve vitamin-filled liquid for homemade soups). Combine with other ingredients and pour into a greased 2-quart baking dish. Bake for 30 minutes.

ZUCCHINI CASSEROLE

Zucchini
Pesto Sauce*
White cheese

Oven 375°

Cut peeled (if zucchini is waxed) or unpeeled zucchini into 3-inch lengths. Split each piece lengthwise. Place in a saucepan. Cover with water and cook until just tender. Drain.

In a greased casserole place cooked pieces. Spread each piece with pesto sauce and top each with a slice of white cheese. Heat in oven until cheese has melted, about 5 minutes.

Yellow

BAKED ACORN SQUASH

Acorn squash
Brown sugar
Uncolored butter

Oven 375°

Cut squash in half. Scoop out seeds. Place cut side up in a large casserole dish or pan. Pour hot water around the squash so at least half the squash is standing in water. Cover dish and bake for 1 hour. Remove from water. Drain each piece thoroughly. Serve with a sprinkle of brown sugar and a generous piece of butter in each cavity.

CARROT RING

Serves 6

6 carrots, grated
1 cup cooked rice
4 ounces uncolored cheese,
  grated

⅓ cup minced onion
2 eggs, beaten
Salt and pepper to taste

Oven 350°

Bring grated carrots to a boil in salted water. Turn to simmer for 5 minutes. Remove from heat and drain. Combine with other ingredients. Pour into oiled 1½-quart ring mold. Bake in a pan of hot water for 30 minutes. Turn out onto platter. Fill center with peas, either plain or creamed.

CORN PANCAKES

Serves 4

1 cup canned or fresh corn
1 egg, well beaten
1 tablespoon pure
  vegetable oil

¼ cup unbleached flour
Salt and pepper to taste

Combine all ingredients and mix well. Drop by spoonfuls onto greased skillet. When brown turn with spatula and brown other side. Serve with Maple Syrup I* or II.*

CORN PUDDING

Serves 5 or 6

3 eggs, slightly beaten
1½ tablespoons pure
   vegetable oil
1 tablespoon sugar
1½ teaspoons salt
¼ teaspoon pepper
1 small onion, finely
   chopped

1 16-ounce can
   cream-style corn
⅓ cup Soft Bread Crumbs*
1 cup milk, scalded
Paprika

Oven 350°

In a large bowl combine all the ingredients except the paprika. Fill a well-greased 1½-quart casserole or soufflé dish with mixture and sprinkle top with paprika. Place in a large pan of hot water and bake for 1¾ hours. Test for doneness by inserting knife in the middle. If knife comes out clean, the pudding is done.

Potatoes, Noodles, and Rice

AU GRATIN POTATOES

Serves 4

2 tablespoons pure
   vegetable oil
2 tablespoons unbleached
   flour
1 cup milk
½ teaspoon salt

1 tablespoon minced chives
1 cup grated white cheese
2 cups cooked diced
   potatoes
Paprika

Oven 375°

In a heavy saucepan mix oil and flour. Stir in milk and continue stirring until sauce comes to a boil. Add salt, chives, and ½ cup grated cheese. Stir until cheese has melted.

Place potatoes in a greased 1½-quart casserole dish. Pour sauce over them and stir gently until potatoes are well coated.

Spread ½ cup grated cheese on top. Sprinkle paprika over cheese for flavor and color. Bake 15 minutes or until top is bubbling.

BOILED BAKED POTATOES

Serves 4 to 6

12 to 18 small potatoes, peeled
½ cup pure vegetable oil
2 tablespoons chopped chives

Oven 500°

Boil potatoes in salted water. Drain, cool, and store in refrigerator. When ready to serve, arrange in shallow baking dish. Cover with oil and sprinkle with chives. Bake for about 10 minutes or until brown.

HOT POTATO SALAD

Serves 6 to 8

8 medium potatoes
2 cups cubed sharp
   uncolored cheese
½ cup chopped onion

1 cup Mayonnaise*
Salt to taste
⅓ cup sliced green olives

Oven 350°

Scrub potatoes, place in a large pan, and cover with water. Cook until tender. Drain and cool. Peel and cube potatoes. Add cheese, onion, mayonnaise, and salt. Toss lightly. Place in a 13×9-inch baking pan. Sprinkle the sliced olives on top. Cover with foil and bake 1 hour.

MACARONI AND CHEESE

Serves 6

1 cup uncooked macaroni
2 tablespoons pure
vegetable oil
2 tablespoons unbleached
flour

1 cup milk
1 teaspoon salt
1½ cups grated sharp
uncolored cheese
Paprika

Oven 350°

Cook macaroni according to package directions. Drain and place in greased 2-quart casserole dish. In a heavy saucepan mix oil and flour and slowly add milk. Stir until sauce thickens. Add salt and 1 cup cheese. Stir until cheese is melted. Pour over macaroni. Top with remaining cheese. Sprinkle with paprika. Bake for 15 minutes.

NOODLES ROMANOFF

Serves 8

1 8-ounce package noodles
1 12-ounce carton cottage
cheese (small curd)
1 8-ounce carton sour
cream
¾ teaspoon instant minced
onion

¾ teaspoon dried parsley
flakes
½ teaspoon salt
Dash of pepper

Cook noodles in boiling salted water according to package directions. Drain and rinse. In a large saucepan combine noodles, cottage cheese, and sour cream. Stir constantly over low heat until mixture is hot. Add onion, parsley, salt, and pepper. Continue to stir over low heat for 2 minutes.

PARMESAN POTATOES

Serves 6

2 9-ounce packages frozen
  French fried potatoes
2 tablespoons melted
  uncolored butter

1 teaspoon onion salt
Paprika
½ cup grated Parmesan
  cheese

Arrange potatoes in a single layer in a shallow baking pan. Brush with melted butter. Sprinkle with onion salt and paprika. Bake as directed on package. When done, sprinkle with cheese, shaking pan to coat potatoes evenly. Serve immediately.

SCALLOPED POTATOES

Serves 6

6 medium potatoes, pared
  and sliced
4 teaspoons instant minced
  onion

2 teaspoons salt
¼ cup unbleached flour
¼ cup uncolored butter
1 to 2 cups milk, warmed

Oven 350°

Grease a 1½-quart baking dish. Put a layer of sliced potatoes in bottom of dish. Sprinkle 1 teaspoon onion, ½ teaspoon salt, 1 tablespoon flour, and 1 tablespoon butter on potatoes. Make four layers of potatoes and other ingredients until dish is full. Pour warm milk over potatoes so that they are almost completely covered. Bake for 1 hour 15 minutes or until potatoes are completely cooked.

SEASONED RICE

Serves 6

1 cup uncooked rice (not quick cooking)

2 cups Chicken Stock or Beef Stock*

1 teaspoon salt

½ teaspoon thyme

½ teaspoon dried parsley flakes

1 tablespoon instant minced onion

1 tablespoon uncolored butter

Combine all ingredients in a heavy saucepan. Bring to a boil. Stir well. Cover and cook over low heat for 20 to 25 minutes or until rice is tender and liquid is absorbed.

Others

BAKED BEANS

Serves 5 to 6

1 cup dry navy beans

3 cups water

¼ teaspoon parsley flakes

1 stalk celery with leaves

1 small bay leaf

1 teaspoon instant minced onion

¼ cup unbleached flour.

½ teaspoon salt

½ cup Chicken or Beef Stock or Broth*

2 tablespoons brown sugar

¼ teaspoon paprika

½ cup water

Oven 350°

Soak beans in water overnight. Drain. Combine beans, water, parsley, celery, bay leaf, onion, and salt in a large saucepan. Bring to a boil. Simmer 2 hours. Beans should be mealy and tender.

Drain beans. Add stock or broth, brown sugar, and paprika. Mix and bake for 15 minutes or until thoroughly heated. Make a paste of water and flour and add as needed to thicken.

BAKED ONIONS

Serves 8

4 large Bermuda onions,
  peeled and cut in half
4 tablespoons uncolored
  butter

¼ cup honey
2 tablespoons water
1 teaspoon paprika
½ teaspoon salt

Oven 350°

Place onions cut side up in a baking pan. Prepare sauce by melting butter with honey in a saucepan. Stir in water, paprika, and salt. Pour mixture over onions. Cover. Bake 1½ hours. Baste several times during baking. Before serving, sprinkle more paprika on onions if desired.

EGGPLANT ITALIANO

Serves 4

1 medium eggplant
⅓ cup milk
½ cup Dry Bread
  Crumbs*
⅓ cup pure vegetable oil
1 cup shredded mozzarella
  cheese

1 teaspoon oregano
¾ cup Pesto Sauce*
⅓ cup grated Parmesan
  cheese

Oven 350°

Wash the eggplant and slice into ½-inch rounds. Dip each slice into milk and then into bread crumbs. In a skillet brown lightly in the oil. Remove from skillet and put eggplant into 1½-quart casserole, overlapping the slices if necessary. Sprinkle shredded mozzarella cheese and oregano over the eggplant and pour the pesto sauce over all. Top with Parmesan cheese. Bake in oven for 20 to 25 minutes until cheese starts to brown.

10

Desserts

Most of your desserts will have to be homemade. Many of these can be made in quantity and tucked in the lunch box, used as an occasional snack treat, or frozen for future use. For instance, you may wish to keep a supply of cupcakes frozen so that you can easily send one to school if there's going to be a party or if your child is asked to a friend's birthday party. On the other hand, you may decide it's better just to let him enjoy the treat everyone else is sharing and hope for the best.

Don't forget simple, nutritious desserts like fresh fruits or homemade gelatin molds with fruit. There are lots of non-salicylate fruits your family will enjoy—blueberries, grapefruits, papayas, pineapples, bananas, and pears to mention a few.

Be sure to avoid the following:

> Prepared cake mixes, piecrusts, and icings
> Prepared pie fillings
> Bleached flour
> Chocolate, at least in the beginning of the diet
> Artificial vanilla or other artificial extracts
> Almonds
> Salicylate fruits
> Colored butter or margarine
> Rinds of citrus fruits, if waxed
> Limeade if it contains artificial coloring
> Colored cheeses

Cakes

CAROB CAKE

Makes 2-8-inch layers

½ cup uncolored butter, softened

1¾ cups packed brown sugar

2 eggs

½ cup carob powder

½ cup water

2½ cups sifted unbleached flour

1 teaspoon baking soda

1 teaspoon salt

⅔ cup buttermilk

2 teaspoons pure vanilla extract

⅔ cup chopped nuts (optional)

Oven 350°

Cream butter and sugar well. Add eggs, beating until fluffy. Blend carob powder with water. Stir into butter and egg mixture. Combine dry ingredients. Add to creamed mixture alternately with the buttermilk, beating well. Add vanilla and nuts. Mix thoroughly. Bake in two 8-inch greased and floured layer cake pans for 30 to 35 minutes. Cool on wire racks. Ice with desired frosting.

CARROT CAKE

Serves 10 to 12

2 cups unbleached flour

2 cups sugar

2 teaspoons baking powder

2 teaspoons baking soda

1 teaspoon cinnamon

1½ cups pure vegetable oil

3 eggs

2 cups packed grated carrots

1 cup undrained sweetened crushed pineapple

½ cup chopped walnuts

Oven 350°

In a large mixing bowl combine dry ingredients. Add oil and eggs and beat until smooth. Stir in carrots, pineapple, and nuts and mix thoroughly. Pour into a greased 9×13×2-inch cake pan and bake for 50 minutes. Cool and ice with Butter Frosting.*

CUPCAKES

Makes 16 cupcakes

1½ cups sifted unbleached
  flour
1 tablespoon baking
  powder
½ teaspoon salt
¼ cup uncolored butter,
  softened

¾ cup sugar
⅔ cup milk
2 eggs, separated
1½ teaspoons pure vanilla
  extract

Oven 350°

In a bowl combine sifted flour, baking powder, and salt. Sift these ingredients again. Set aside. In a large mixing bowl combine butter with sugar, milk, egg yolks, and vanilla. Beat until well combined. Add flour mixture slowly. Beat for 2 minutes. Whip egg whites until stiff. Carefully fold egg whites into batter and mix thoroughly. Spoon batter into paper-lined cupcake pans, filling about two-thirds full. Bake for 20 to 25 minutes or until top springs back when lightly touched. Frost when completely cooled.

DESSERT ROLL

Serves 6

Cake

4 eggs, separated
¼ cup milk
1 cup sugar
1 cup sifted unbleached
  flour

¼ teaspoon salt
1 teaspoon baking powder
1 teaspoon pure vanilla
  extract

Filling

1 cup pure whipping cream
⅓ cup sugar
1 tablespoon cocoa or
   carob powder

Oven 350°

In a small mixing bowl, beat together egg yolks, milk, and sugar for several minutes until very light and fluffy. Combine flour, salt, and baking powder and slowly add to egg mixture. In a separate bowl, beat egg whites until stiff. While continuing to beat add the vanilla and the egg and flour batter. Beat for an additional 3 to 4 minutes on medium speed. Prepare a 15×10×1-inch jelly roll pan by lining with aluminum foil and grease. Pour batter into pan and bake for 12 to 15 minutes until lightly browned. Remove from oven and immediately turn cake out onto a piece of foil which has been generously dusted with confectioners' sugar. Remove the top foil. Cut crisp edges off the cake and roll together with foil from narrow end. Allow the cake to cool completely.

When ready to fill, whip cream with sugar and cocoa until stiff. Unroll cake and spread with cream filling. Reroll and sift confectioners' sugar on top. Chill until ready to serve.

EASY CAROB CAKE (EGGLESS)

Makes 1 8-inch square cake
or 16 cupcakes

1½ cups sifted unbleached
   flour
1 cup sugar
1 teaspoon baking soda
½ teaspoon salt
2 tablespoons carob
   powder

1 teaspoon pure vanilla
   extract
1 tablespoon white distilled
   vinegar
5 tablespoons uncolored
   butter, melted
1 cup water

Oven 350°

Combine all dry ingredients together. Add vanilla, vinegar, and melted butter. Mix well. Stir in water and mix until all ingredients are thoroughly blended. Bake in a greased 8-inch-square pan 40 to 45 minutes or until a toothpick inserted in the center comes out clean. Cool in pan 10 minutes. Remove and cool thoroughly on wire rack. May be iced.

To make cupcakes, fill sixteen cupcake liners two-thirds full with batter. Bake at 375° for 15 minutes or until a toothpick inserted in the center comes out clean.

EASY GINGERBREAD (EGGLESS)

Makes 1 8- or 9-inch square cake
or 18 cupcakes

1 cup pure molasses
 (whatever type you
 prefer)
½ cup packed brown sugar
½ cup melted uncolored
 butter or pure vegetable
 oil
¾ teaspoon cinnamon

¾ teaspoon nutmeg
1 teaspoon ginger
½ cup boiling water
2½ cups unsifted
 unbleached flour
1 teaspoon baking soda
Granulated sugar

Oven 350°

Combine molasses, brown sugar, butter, and spices. Stir in boiling water. Mix in flour. Add baking soda and stir until thoroughly mixed. Pour into well-greased 8- or 9-inch square cake pan. Sprinkle top with granulated sugar. Bake 30 to 35 minutes or until a toothpick inserted in the center comes out clean. Serve warm, with Lemon Sauce* or Whipped Topping* if desired. Rewarm leftovers or serve cold. Great for snacks and lunch boxes. If making cupcakes, fill pans two-thirds full. Bake at 375° about 15 minutes.

SNACK-TIME SPARKLES

Serves 8

Cake recipe from Dessert Roll*

Icing

1 cup sugar
¼ cup light corn syrup
2 tablespoons water

2 egg whites
½ teaspoon pure vanilla
  extract

Oven 350°

Prepare cake batter as directed for dessert roll. Take eight paper cups (the type used for hot coffee but not styrofoam) and oil and dust the insides with confectioners' sugar. Place on a cookie sheet and divide the cake batter evenly into the cups. Bake for 20 to 25 minutes or until lightly browned. Allow to cool completely.

To prepare icing, combine sugar, syrup, water, and egg whites in top of a double boiler. Place over simmering water and beat with electric mixer on medium-high speed about 10 to 12 minutes until stiff peaks form. Remove from heat and stir in vanilla.

When ready to fill cakes, run a sharp knife around the cakes and remove from the cups. Split and fill. The cakes can be put back into the paper cups and are then easily packed in a lunch box.

Makes a delicious substitute for store-bought cream-filled spongecake.

PINEAPPLE OR BLUEBERRY UPSIDE-DOWN CAKE OR CUPCAKES

Makes 1 9-inch round cake
or 15 cupcakes

Basic Cake

1 egg	¼ teaspoon salt
¾ cup sugar	¼ cup uncolored butter,
1 cup sifted unbleached	melted
flour	½ cup milk
1½ teaspoons baking	1 teaspoon pure vanilla
powder	extract

Pineapple Topping

½ cup packed brown sugar	1 cup well-drained
3 tablespoons uncolored	unsweetened crushed
butter, melted	pineapple
2 tablespoons pineapple	
juice	

Blueberry Topping

½ cup sugar	½ cup fresh, canned (well
3 tablespoons uncolored	drained) or frozen
butter, melted	(thawed) blueberries
2 tablespoons pineapple	
juice or water	

Oven 350°

To prepare the cake batter beat egg and sugar together with an electric mixer. In another bowl combine all dry ingredients. Add butter, milk, and vanilla. Beat for 1 minute. Add egg and sugar mixture and continue beating for another minute.

To prepare either topping, stir sugar into melted butter until dissolved. Add juice or water and mix well. If making a cake, spread butter and sugar mixture over entire bottom of 9-inch round cake pan. Evenly distribute fruit on top. Pour cake batter on top. Bake for 35 to 40 minutes or until cake pulls away from sides of pan. Let cool for 5 minutes. Turn upside down onto a plate, but do not remove pan for another 5 minutes.

If making cupcakes, divide butter and sugar mixture among fifteen cupcake liners. Distribute fruit evenly. Pour cake on top. Bake at 375° for about 20 minutes. Let cool before removing from cupcake liners.

To pack in a lunch box, wrap well and pack with a plastic spoon.

MOCK APPLESAUCE CAKE (PEARS)

Makes 1 8×8-inch square cake

½ cup uncolored butter, softened
1 cup sugar
1 egg, slightly beaten
1½ cups Mock Applesauce*

2 cups unsifted unbleached flour
1½ teaspoons cinnamon
½ teaspoon nutmeg
1 teaspoon baking soda
1 cup chopped nuts

Oven 350°

Cream butter and sugar together. Add egg and mock applesauce. Mix well. Stir in dry ingredients. Beat well, using an electric mixer for several minutes. Stir in chopped nuts. Pour into a greased and floured 8×8-inch cake pan. Bake for 60 to 65 minutes or until a toothpick inserted in the center comes out clean. Serve plain, with Lemon Sauce* or frost with desired icing.

BUTTER FROSTING

Makes 2 cups frosting or frosts
1 8- or 9-inch layer cake

¼ cup uncolored butter, softened
1 1-pound package confectioners' sugar, unsifted

¼ teaspoon salt
1 tablespoon pure vanilla extract
¼ cup milk or light cream

Cream together butter, sugar, salt, and vanilla. Add milk slowly until desired spreading consistency is reached.

LEMON FROSTING

Makes 2 cups frosting or frosts
1 8- or 9-inch layer cake

Butter Frosting*
2 tablespoons pure lemon juice

Prepare lemon frosting as directed above in butter frosting, substituting lemon juice for vanilla.

CAROB FROSTING

Makes 2 cups frosting or frosts
1 8- or 9-inch layer cake

Butter Frosting*
2 to 4 tablespoons sifted carob powder

Prepare carob frosting as directed in butter frosting above, mixing in carob powder until thoroughly blended.

FLUFFY ICING

Makes enough icing for
1 8- or 9-inch cake

1 cup sugar
¼ cup light corn syrup
2 tablespoons water

2 egg whites
½ teaspoon pure vanilla extract

In the top of a double boiler mix together sugar, corn syrup, water, and egg whites. Place over simmering water and beat with an electric mixer on medium-high speed for 10 to 12 minutes until stiff peaks form. Remove from heat and blend in vanilla.

CAROB OR CHOCOLATE FLUFFY ICING

Combine 2 tablespoons carob powder or cocoa with the Fuffy Icing* recipe. Mix as indicated above.

Brownies and Squares

BUTTERSCOTCH BROWNIES

Makes 32 2-inch squares

1½ cups packed brown
   sugar
½ cup uncolored butter,
   melted
2 eggs, slightly beaten
1 teaspoon pure vanilla
   extract

1½ cups unbleached flour
2 teaspoons baking powder
½ teaspoon salt
½ to 1 cup chopped nuts
   or dates

Oven 350°

Add sugar to melted butter. Stir until sugar dissolves. Cool. Add eggs and vanilla and beat until creamy. Add dry ingredients and mix well. Fold in nuts or dates. Divide batter in half. Pour each half into a well-greased 8-inch-square pan. Smooth batter into corners with spoon. Bake 20 to 25 minutes until toothpick inserted into center comes out clean. Cool. Cut into squares. May be frozen. Great for lunch box.

CAROB FUDGE BROWNIES

Makes 16 brownies

⅔ cup sifted unbleached
   flour
½ teaspoon baking powder
¼ teaspoon salt
¼ cup sifted carob powder
⅓ cup uncolored butter,
   melted

1 cup packed brown sugar
2 eggs, well beaten
1 teaspoon pure vanilla
   extract
½ cup chopped nuts

Oven 350°

Combine flour, baking powder, and salt and sift together. Add carob powder to melted butter. Add the sugar gradually to eggs, beating thoroughly. Blend carob mixture with eggs and sugar. Add flour and blend thoroughly. Stir in vanilla and nuts and mix well. Spread in a buttered 8-inch-square pan. Bake 25 minutes. Cool. Cut in squares.

CHOCOLATE BROWNIES

Makes 24 squares

3 squares (3 ounces)
  unsweetened chocolate
½ cup uncolored butter
1¾ cups sugar
3 eggs
1¼ cups unbleached flour
1½ teaspoons baking
  powder

1 teaspoon salt
1 teaspoon pure vanilla
  extract
¾ cup chopped nuts
  (optional)

Oven 350°

In top of double boiler melt the three squares of chocolate and butter, stirring occasionally. Remove from heat. Beat in sugar and eggs. In a separate bowl combine flour, baking powder, and salt. Stir dry ingredients into the chocolate mixture and add vanilla and nuts. Spread the batter in a greased 13×9×2-inch pan and bake for 30 minutes. Cool in pan and cut into squares.

LEMON TREATS

Makes 12 squares

1 cup uncolored butter
½ cup powdered sugar
2 cups unbleached flour
4 eggs
5 tablespoons pure lemon
  juice

2 cups sugar
4 tablespoons unbleached
  flour
1 teaspoon baking powder
½ teaspoon salt

Oven 350°

Place butter in a 9×13×2-inch pan and put in oven while preheating until completely melted. Remove pan from oven and add the powdered sugar and 2 cups flour. Mix thoroughly and press firmly into the bottom of the pan. Bake in the oven for 20 minutes. While crust is baking, mix the remaining ingredients and beat for several minutes until very light and fluffy. Pour this mixture on top of the hot crust and return to the oven for an additional 25 minutes. Remove and immediately sift additional powdered sugar on top. Can be served warm or cold.

PINEAPPLE NUT SQUARES

Makes 16 2-inch squares

1⅓ cups sifted unbleached flour
½ teaspoon baking powder
¼ teaspoon salt
1¼ cups packed brown sugar
¼ cup pure vegetable oil
2 eggs

¾ cup drained sweetened crushed pineapple, reserve liquid
2 tablespoons pineapple syrup
½ teaspoon pure vanilla extract
½ cup chopped nuts

Oven 350°

Combine flour, baking powder, salt, and sugar. Add remaining ingredients and mix thoroughly. Pour into a greased 8-inch-square pan. Bake for 35 to 40 minutes until slightly browned. Cool and cut into squares.

Crusts

PIECRUST

Makes single pastry for 8- or 9-inch pie

1 cup plus 2 tablespoons unsifted unbleached flour

¾ teaspoon salt
⅓ cup pure vegetable oil
2 tablespoons milk

Oven 450°

Mix flour and salt together in a bowl. In a cup measure oil and milk but do not mix. Add to the flour mixture. Stir until well mixed. With your hands form a smooth ball. Place on a sheet of waxed paper and flatten a little. Cover with another sheet of waxed paper and roll out with a rolling pin to desired size and thickness. Peel off top paper. With paper on top of dough place in pie pan and carefully peel off paper. Fit into pan and press dough around edges. If baking only the crust, prick in several spots with a fork. Bake for 10 to 12 minutes, or until lightly browned. Double recipe for a two-crust pie.

GRAHAM CRACKER PIECRUST

Makes crust
for 8- or 9-inch pie

1½ cups Graham Cracker*
  crumbs
½ cup uncolored butter,
  melted

⅓ cup confectioners' sugar
1 teaspoon cinnamon
  (optional)

Mix cracker crumbs with butter, sugar, and cinnamon. Pat firmly into pie pan. May be baked at 350° for 5 to 7 minutes. Chill. Fill with any desired filling. Especially good for ice cream pies.

CORN FLAKE CRUST

Makes crust
for 8- or 9-inch pie

1 cup crushed additive-free
  corn flakes
¼ cup uncolored butter,
  melted

3 tablespoons sugar
1½ teaspoons cinnamon

Mix together all ingredients. Press mixture in bottom of pan to form crust. May be baked at 350° for 5 minutes.

GINGER SNAP CRUST

Makes crust for
8-inch round or square pie

1½ cups Ginger Snap* crumbs
⅓ cup uncolored butter, melted

Make the Ginger Snap crumbs by putting the cookies through a blender or grinder. Melt the butter in the bottom of an 8-inch-square or 8-inch-round cake pan and blend in the cookie crumbs with a fork until crumbly. Press against the sides and bottom of the pan to form crust.

Pies

BLUEBERRY PIE

Makes 1 8- or 9-inch pie

Double recipe Piecrust*
4 cups fresh, canned or
frozen (thawed)
blueberries
1 tablespoon water
1 tablespoon pure lemon
juice

1 cup sugar
4 to 5 tablespoons
unbleached flour
2 tablespoons uncolored
butter

Oven 375°

Prepare piecrusts. Combine berries, water, lemon juice, and sugar in a heavy saucepan. Cook over medium heat until berries are tender. Add flour. Stir until filling thickens. Cool. Pour into prepared pie shell. Dot with butter. Cover with top crust. Slit top crust with knife in several places. Bake for about 30 minutes or until crust is golden brown.

BLUEBERRY TURNOVERS

Makes 10 to 12 small or
5 to 6 large turnovers

1 cup fresh, canned, or
frozen (thawed)
blueberries
2 tablespoons water or
juice from berries
¼ cup sugar

1 teaspoon pure lemon
juice
1 tablespoon cornstarch
mixed with 1 tablespoon
cold water
1 recipe Piecrust*

Oven 425°

Combine blueberries, water, sugar, and lemon juice in a saucepan. Cook until blueberries are tender. Add cornstarch mixed with water to thicken filling. Continue cooking until filling is thick.

Roll out piecrust between waxed paper as thin as possible. Cut into squares or circles. Put small amount of filling on piecrust. Fold over. Seal edges by pressing them together. Prick top of each with a fork.

Place on a greased cookie sheet. Bake for 10 to 12 minutes until lightly browned. Serve hot or cold. May be frozen.

BLUEBERRY-CRANBERRY PIE

Makes 1 8- or 9-inch pie

Double recipe Piecrust*
2 cups fresh, canned, or
frozen (thawed)
blueberries
1½ cups fresh or frozen
(thawed) cranberries
1½ cups sugar

¼ cup hot water
¼ cup cornstarch
¼ teaspoon pure lemon
extract
¼ teaspoon salt
2 tablespoons uncolored
butter

Oven 425°

Prepare piecrusts. In a heavy saucepan, combine berries, sugar, and hot water. Bring to a boil, stirring frequently. Reduce heat and cook until berries are tender. Add cornstarch, lemon extract, and salt and stir until filling thickens. Pour into a pie shell. Dot butter over filling. Cover with top crust. Slit crust in several places to allow steam to escape. Bake for about 8 minutes. Reduce heat to 325° and bake for 35 to 40 minutes or until crust is lightly browned.

ICE CREAM PIE

Graham Cracker Piecrust* or Ginger Snap Crust*
½ gallon "safe" ice cream, one or more flavors

Prepare crust. Soften ice cream and fill pie shell. Freeze until firm. If using several flavors, soften one at a time, spread in pie shell, freeze, soften another, and spread on top of first frozen layer. Vanilla, lemon, and carob ice creams make a good combination.

INDIVIDUAL MERINGUES

Makes 4 meringues

2 egg whites
⅛ teaspoon cream of
  tartar

½ cup sugar
½ teaspoon pure vanilla
  extract

Oven 225°

Beat egg whites with an electric mixer until they begin to foam. Add cream of tartar and beat until very stiff. Add sugar very gradually, beating constantly. Add vanilla and beat into mixture.

Cover a cookie sheet with plain brown paper. Brown paper from a grocery bag works well. With a large spoon make four mounds of beaten mixture on brown paper. Make a hollow in each mound with a spoon. Bake for 1 hour. Turn off heat, open oven door part way so meringues will cool very slowly. While they are still warm, press gently in the middle of each to break the crust if you wish to fill them later with a cream filling or ice cream. May be stored at room temperature for several days.

LEMON ICE CREAM PIE

Makes 1 8- or 9-inch pie

1 quart "safe" vanilla ice cream
3 ounces frozen "safe" lemonade concentrate
1 8- or 9-inch Ginger Snap Crust,* Graham Cracker
   Piecrust,* or Corn Flake Crust*

Soften ice cream. Mix thoroughly with the lemonade concentrate. Fill prepared crust. Cover and store in freezer.

LIME CHIFFON PIE

Makes 1 8- or 9-inch pie

1 envelope unflavored
   gelatin
½ cup water
¾ cup sugar
⅓ cup pure lime juice

3 eggs, separated
¼ teaspoon cream of
   tartar
1 recipe Piecrust*

Combine gelatin, water, ½ cup sugar, lime juice, and egg yolks in a medium saucepan and bring to a boil over medium heat, stirring constantly. Chill mixture until it mounds slightly when stirred. Beat egg whites until fluffy. Slowly add ¼ cup sugar and cream of tartar and continue to beat until the whites stand in stiff peaks. Fold the chilled mixture gently into the egg whites and mix thoroughly. Pour into a baked 8- or 9-inch pie crust and refrigerate for several hours until set. May be served topped with whipped cream.

MOCK TART CHERRY PIE (CRANBERRY)

Makes 1 8- or 9-inch pie

3½ cups fresh or frozen
  (thawed) cranberries
¼ cup hot water
2¼ cups sugar
½ teaspoon pure lemon
  extract

4 to 5 tablespoons
  cornstarch
2 egg yolks, slightly beaten
Double recipe Piecrust*
2 tablespoons uncolored
  butter

Oven 425°

In a heavy saucepan combine cranberries, water, and sugar. Bring to a boil and continue cooking until berries are tender. Add lemon extract and cornstarch and cook until filling thickens. Remove from heat. Stir in egg yolks. Pour into pie shell. Dot butter over filling. Cover with top crust. Slit crust in several places to allow steam to escape. Bake for about 8 minutes. Reduce heat to 325° and bake for 35 to 40 minutes or until crust is lightly browned.

Tastes and looks a lot like a tart cherry pie.

PEAR PIE

Makes 1 8- or 9-inch pie

Double recipe Piecrust*
5 cups thinly sliced peeled
  fresh pears
¾ cup sugar plus 1
  tablespoon
½ teaspoon cinnamon

¼ teaspoon nutmeg
1½ tablespoons
  unbleached flour
1 tablespoon uncolored
  butter
1 tablespoon milk

Oven 400°

Line 8- or 9-inch pie pan with bottom pastry. Toss pears lightly with ¾ cup sugar, cinnamon, nutmeg, and flour. Place pears in crust and dot with butter. Cover with remaining pastry and cut vents in top to let steam escape. Brush top pastry with milk and sprinkle lightly with 1 tablespoon sugar. Bake for 30 to 40 minutes until crust is lightly browned. Cool before serving.

PECAN PIE

Makes 1 8- or 9-inch pie

Makes 1 8- or 9-inch pie

⅓ cup uncolored butter,
   softened
¾ cup sugar
3 eggs
¾ cup light corn syrup

½ teaspoon pure vanilla
   extract
¼ teaspoon salt
1 cup broken pieces pecans
1 recipe Piecrust*

Oven 350°

In a large mixing bowl cream butter and sugar with an electric mixer. Add one egg at a time, beating constantly. Stir in corn syrup, vanilla, and salt. Blend well and add pecans. Pour into unbaked 8- or 9-inch pie shell. Bake for 50 minutes or until a knife inserted in the center comes out clean.

PUMPKIN PIE

Makes 1 8- or 9-inch pie

½ cup packed brown sugar
1 tablespoon unbleached
   flour
½ teaspoon salt
1½ teaspoons cinnamon
½ teaspoon nutmeg

½ teaspoon ginger
2 eggs
1½ cups pumpkin
1½ cups evaporated milk
1 recipe Piecrust*

Oven 375°

In a small bowl combine sugar, flour, salt, cinnamon, nutmeg, and ginger. Set aside. Beat eggs until light and fluffy. Add pumpkin and mix well. Stir in dry ingredients. Gradually add milk and stir until mixed thoroughly. Pour into unbaked 8- or 9-inch piecrust. Bake for 45 to 55 minutes or until a knife blade will come out clean when inserted in center of filling.

QUICK LEMON MERINGUE PIE

Makes 1 8- or 9-inch pie

½ cup pure lemon juice
1⅓ cups sweetened
   condensed milk

2 egg yolks
1 recipe Piecrust*
Meringue Topping*

Oven 325°

In a mixing bowl beat together lemon juice and condensed milk. Add egg yolks and beat until well blended. Pour into baked 8- or 9-inch piecrust. Prepare meringue topping. Pile lightly on pie filling and spread out completely to cover the filling. Bake until lightly browned, about 15 to 20 minutes.

MERINGUE TOPPING

Makes topping for 1 pie

¼ teaspoon cream of tartar
2 egg whites
¼ cup sugar

Oven 325°

In a mixing bowl combine cream of tartar and egg whites. Beat until almost thick enough to hold a peak. Add sugar gradually, beating until stiff but not dry. Pile lightly on pie filling and spread out to cover. Bake for 15 to 20 minutes.

RHUBARB PIE

Makes 1 8- or 9-inch pie

Double recipe Piecrust*
4 cups 1-inch pieces fresh
   or frozen (thawed)
   rhubarb
1⅔ cups sugar
¼ cup unbleached flour

⅛ teaspoon salt
⅛ teaspoon nutmeg
1 teaspoon pure lemon
   juice
Uncolored butter

Oven 400°

Prepare piecrust. In a large mixing bowl combine rhubarb, sugar, flour, salt, nutmeg, and lemon juice. Mix well. Pour into pie shell. Dot with butter. Top with lattice crust. Bake for 50 to 60 minutes or until crust is golden brown.

VANILLA CREAM PIE

Makes 8- or 9-inch pie

3 tablespoons cornstarch
⅔ cup sugar
½ teaspoon salt
2⅓ cups milk
2 egg yolks, slightly beaten

1 tablespoon pure vegetable oil
1½ teaspoons pure vanilla extract
1 recipe Piecrust*

In a heavy saucepan combine cornstarch, sugar, and salt. Add milk. Stir constantly over medium heat until sauce comes to a boil. Stir 1 minute longer. Remove from heat and very slowly pour in egg yolks, stirring vigorously. Add oil and vanilla and blend well. Cover and cool. Pour into baked 8- or 9-inch piecrust. Chill thoroughly. May be served with whipped cream or with Meringue Topping.*

BANANA CREAM PIE

Makes 1 8- or 9-inch pie

Cover baked 8- or 9-inch piecrust with 2 medium sliced bananas. Pour Vanilla Cream Pie* filling on top and bake with Meringue Topping* or chill and serve plain or with whipped cream.

11
Pudding and
Frozen Desserts

Puddings are easily prepared from scratch without much fuss. They may be included in lunch boxes by placing them in a wide-mouth thermos—include a plastic spoon. Ice creams are delicious, easy, and fun for the whole family to make. Be sure to make lots as it won't last long. A scoop of ice cream in a thermos of milk will brighten up any lunch.

Avoid the following:

> Bleached flour
> Salicylate fruits
> Prepared pudding or gelatin mixes
> Chocolate, at least in the beginning of the diet
> Colored butter or margarine

Puddings

VANILLA PUDDING

Serves 6

½ cup sugar
¼ cup cornstarch
¼ teaspoon salt
2⅔ cups milk

2 tablespoons uncolored butter
1 teaspoon pure vanilla extract

In a large saucepan combine sugar, cornstarch, and salt. Add milk slowly and stir until smooth. Cook over medium heat, stirring constantly while mixture boils. Continue stirring and boil 1 minute longer. Remove from heat. Stir in butter and vanilla and mix well. Refrigerate in a covered container.

CAROB OR CHOCOLATE PUDDING

Serves 6

Vanilla Pudding*
2 squares unsweetened chocolate or 2 to 4 tablespoons carob powder

Prepare vanilla pudding as directed. Add chocolate or carob powder when vanilla is added. Stir until well mixed and chocolate or carob is melted. Refrigerate in a covered container.

BUTTERSCOTCH PUDDING

Serves 6

2 tablespoons uncolored butter   ½ cup water
⅔ cup packed brown sugar   Vanilla Pudding*

In a large saucepan stir and melt butter and brown sugar over low heat. Add water and cook until mixture is smooth. Set aside. Prepare vanilla pudding. When cooking is completed add butterscotch mixture and mix well. Refrigerate in a covered container.

LEMON PUDDING

Serves 6

Vanilla Pudding*
6 tablespoons pure lemon juice

Prepare vanilla pudding as directed. Substitute lemon juice for vanilla extract.

PINEAPPLE PUDDING

Serves 6

Vanilla Pudding*
⅔ cup drained crushed unsweetened pineapple
2 tablespoons pure lemon juice

Prepare vanilla pudding as directed. Substitute lemon juice for vanilla extract and fold in crushed pineapple.

Frozen Desserts

LEMON ICE CREAM

Makes ½ gallon or
8 to 10 servings

1⅓ cups sweetened
  condensed milk
1 cup water
2 teaspoons pure vanilla
  extract

½ cup pure lemon juice
1 teaspoon pure lemon
  extract
2 cups (1 pint) heavy cream

Combine condensed milk, water, vanilla, lemon juice, and lemon extract in a large bowl. Chill. Whip heavy cream until slightly thickened. Fold into chilled condensed milk mixture. Pour into 8×8-inch pans. Freeze until almost firm, about 2 hours. Place in a large, chilled mixing bowl and beat with an electric mixer until smooth. Return to pans, individual paper cups, or other molds. Cover with foil and freeze until firm.

VANILLA ICE CREAM I

Makes ½ gallon or
Serves 8 to 10

1⅓ cups sweetened
  condensed milk
1 cup water

1 tablespoon pure vanilla
  extract
2 cups whipping cream

Combine condensed milk, water, and vanilla. Chill. Whip heavy cream until slightly thickened. Fold into chilled condensed milk mixture. Pour into 8×8-inch pans. Freeze until almost firm, about 2 hours. Place in a large, chilled mixing bowl and beat with an electric mixer until smooth. Return to pans, individual paper cups, or other molds. Cover with foil and freeze until firm.

CAROB OR CHOCOLATE ICE CREAM I

Makes ½ gallon or
Serves 8 to 10

Vanilla Ice Cream I*
½ to ¾ cup sifted carob powder or ¼ to ½ cup cocoa

Prepare ice cream as above for vanilla ice cream but dissolve carob powder or cocoa in hot condensed milk in the top of a double boiler before adding water and vanilla. Then chill.

VANILLA ICE CREAM II

Serves 8

1 envelope unflavored
  gelatin
2 cups cold milk (regular
  or 2 per cent)
2 eggs, separated
⅔ cup sugar

⅛ teaspoon salt
2 teaspoons pure vanilla
  extract
2 cups (1 pint) half and
  half cream

Sprinkle gelatin over cold milk in top of double boiler. Place over boiling water and stir until gelatin is dissolved. Cool. Add egg yolks, sugar, and salt. Beat well with an electric mixer. Place again over boiling water and cook, stirring constantly until mixture coats spoon. Remove from heat. Cool. Stir in vanilla and cream. Pour into 8×8-inch pans and freeze until almost firm. Beat egg whites until stiff. Place frozen mixture into chilled bowl and beat until smooth. Fold in egg whites. Return to pans and freeze until firm.

CAROB OR CHOCOLATE ICE CREAM II

Vanilla Ice Cream II*
6 to 8 tablespoons carob powder or cocoa

Prepare ice cream as directed, but dissolve carob powder or cocoa in hot milk containing the dissolved gelatin.

CRANBERRY OR WATERMELON SHERBET

Serves 8 to 10

1 envelope unflavored
  gelatin
½ cup cold water
1 cup sugar
1 cup hot water
2 cups cranberry juice or
  watermelon pulp

1 tablespoon pure lemon
  juice
2 egg whites
¼ teaspoon salt

Sprinkle gelatin over cold water. Set aside. Combine sugar and hot water in saucepan and bring to a full boil. Continue to cook until the syrup reaches the thread stage (230°). If using watermelon pulp, place in blender on low speed for 15 seconds. Remove syrup from heat and stir in softened gelatin, fruit and lemon juice. Chill until the mixture thickens. Whip the egg whites together with the salt until stiff peaks form. Fold gently but thoroughly into the gelatin mixture. Pour into two refrigerator trays and freeze until mushy. Beat the mixture until light and pour back into refrigerator trays. Freeze until firm.

PINEAPPLE FLUFF

Serves 6

1 envelope unflavored
gelatin
¼ cup cold water
3 eggs, separated
1 teaspoon pure lemon
extract
2 tablespoons pure lemon
juice

½ cup sugar
½ teaspoon salt
⅔ cup drained crushed
canned pineapple
½ cup pure whipping
cream

Soften gelatin in cold water. In the top of a double boiler, beat egg yolks. Add lemon extract, lemon juice, sugar, and salt. Cook over boiling water, stirring constantly until mixture thickens and coats spoon. Remove from heat. Add softened gelatin. Stir until dissolved. Add pineapple and refrigerate until mixture begins to thicken. Whip cream. Beat egg whites until stiff. Fold each into pineapple mixture. Refrigerate in a covered container or pour into a 2-quart mold and chill. Or pour into your favorite piecrust. Chill.

PINEAPPLE SUPREME

Serves 4

1 envelope unflavored
gelatin
½ cup cold water
1 tablespoon pure lemon
juice

1 9-ounce can crushed
pineapple, undrained
2 3-ounce packages cream
cheese

Sprinkle gelatin over water in a small saucepan. Dissolve over medium heat, stirring constantly. Stir in lemon juice. In a blender liquefy pineapple with half the cream cheese. When completely blended add the remaining cream cheese and liquefy. Combine with gelatin. Pour into individual dessert dishes. Chill until set.

LEMON DELIGHT DESSERT

Serves 6

1 envelope unflavored
  gelatin
¾ cup sugar
¼ teaspoon salt
3 eggs, separated

⅓ cup pure lemon juice
⅓ cup water
⅓ cup sour cream
¼ cup sugar

In top of a double boiler mix gelatin, sugar, and salt. Beat in egg yolks, lemon juice, and water. Cook over simmering water, stirring constantly for about 10 minutes. When mixture begins to coat spoon remove from stove. Chill until mixture starts to thicken. Stir in sour cream. In a small bowl beat egg whites until they begin to hold their shape. Continue to beat as sugar is added and egg whites become stiff but not dry. Fold egg whites into lemon mixture. Spoon into individual dishes or large bowl and refrigerate.

CAROB MOUSSE

Serves 8 to 10

⅔ cup carob powder
⅓ cup water
¾ cup sugar
¼ teaspoon salt
3 eggs, separated
2 cups pure whipping
  cream

1 teaspoon pure vanilla
  extract
2 cups cut-up
  Marshmallows*
  (optional)

In the top of a double boiler combine carob powder, water, sugar, salt, and slightly beaten egg yolks. Stir well. Cook over boiling water for 3 minutes. Let cool. Whip cream. Beat egg whites until stiff. Add vanilla to carob mixture and fold in cream and egg whites until thoroughly mixed. Fold in marshmallows if desired. Pour into freezer trays and freeze.

Others

COMPANY CHEESE CAKE

Serves 6

1 envelope unflavored
  gelatin
¼ cup cold water
1 egg, separated
¼ cup sugar
½ cup milk
¼ teaspoon salt
1 cup cottage cheese
1 tablespoon pure lemon
  juice

¼ teaspoon pure lemon
  extract
½ cup pure whipping
  cream or evaporated
  milk, chilled and
  whipped
1 recipe Corn Flake Crust*
  or 1 recipe Piecrust,*
  baked

Soften gelatin in cold water. In the top of a double boiler, beat egg yolk slightly, add sugar, milk, and salt. Cook over boiling water until mixture coats the spoon. Add gelatin to custard and stir until dissolved. Place cottage cheese in a blender on highest speed until smooth and creamy. Add cottage cheese, lemon juice, and lemon extract to custard. Cool until custard begins to thicken. Whip cream or evaporated milk and beat egg white until stiff. Fold both into custard.

Prepare corn flake crust or baked piecrust. If using corn flakes, place most of the crumbs in the bottom of an 8- or 9-inch pie pan or 1½-quart mold. Add cheese mixture. Sprinkle remaining crumbs on top and chill thoroughly. Unmold when ready to serve. Or pour cheese mixture into baked pie shell and chill.

EASY CHEESE CAKE

Serves 8

1 recipe Graham Cracker
  Piecrust* or 1 recipe
  Ginger Snap Crust*
2 eight-ounce packages
  cream cheese

2 eggs
½ cup sugar
½ teaspoon pure vanilla
  extract
1 cup sour cream

Oven 350°

Prepare graham cracker piecrust or ginger snap crust and press against sides and bottom of an 8-inch-square pan or 8-inch-round cake pan. In a small mixer bowl beat cream cheese until creamy. Add eggs, sugar, and vanilla and beat until very smooth. Pour into crumb-lined pan and bake for 35 minutes. Remove from oven and immediately spread sour cream evenly on top. Cool and serve. Refrigerate any leftovers.

BAKED PEARS

Serves 3

2 large pears, cored,
  peeled, and cut in sixths
¼ cup honey
¼ cup packed brown sugar
1 tablespoon pure lemon
  juice

¼ teaspoon cinnamon
¼ teaspoon ginger
⅛ teaspoon nutmeg

Oven 350°

Place pears in baking dish. Combine remaining ingredients and pour over pears. Bake 30 to 40 minutes. Pears should be barely tender. Serve slightly warm or cold.

MOCK APPLE CRISP (PEARS)

Serves 4

5 or 6 winter pears, cored,
 peeled, and sliced
½ cup unbleached flour

½ cup sugar
¼ cup uncolored butter,

Oven 375°

Place pear slices in a deep pan or Pyrex dish. Mix together flour, sugar, and butter, working quickly so it does not become oily. Spread on top of the sliced pears. Bake for 30 minutes or until pears are done and the topping is beginning to brown. May be served warm or cold. Good with Whipped Topping,* whipped cream, or a spoonful of ice cream on each portion.

RHUBARB DESSERT

Serves 4

¼ cup uncolored butter,
 melted
¾ cup sugar
1½ cups Dry Bread
 Crumbs*

2 cups finely sliced
 uncooked rhubarb

Oven 325°

Mix together butter, sugar, and bread crumbs. Stir in rhubarb. Place in greased 8×8-inch pan or dish. Bake for 45 minutes. Serve with Whipped Topping,* whipped cream, or ice cream.

STEWED RHUBARB

Makes 1½ cups

3 cups (3 stalks) 1-inch lengths uncooked rhubarb
3 tablespoons water
¼ cup sugar

Place rhubarb and water in a heavy saucepan. Cover and bring to a boil over medium heat. If necessary, add a little more water so rhubarb does not stick to pan. Reduce heat and simmer covered until rhubarb is soft. Add sugar and cook 1 minute longer. Stir well. Cool and refrigerate. Add more sugar if desired.

SPANISH CREAM

Serves 6

3 cups milk
1 envelope unflavored
  gelatin
½ cup sugar
¼ teaspoon salt

3 egg yolks, slightly beaten
1 teaspoon pure vanilla
  extract
3 egg whites, stiffly beaten

Pour milk into top of double boiler. Sprinkle gelatin over milk. Place pan over hot water. Add sugar and salt, stirring until dissolved. Pour slightly beaten egg yolks slowly into milk. Cook until somewhat thickened, stirring constantly. Remove from heat. Add vanilla and allow to cool at room temperature. Fold in stiffly beaten egg whites. Turn into a 1-quart mold or cake pan which has been rinsed in cold water. Chill until set.

12

Snacks and Beverages

If your child is used to a lot of junk foods and soda pop, snack time will seem like a problem at first. Don't despair. There are several types of soda pop available that are uncolored and naturally flavored (see Appendix B). You should realize, however, they do contain other additives. There are many safe fruit juice beverages you can buy which will be very nutritious.

Several brands of crackers should be okay (check Appendix B). You'll probably have to make your own cookies. Popcorn makes an easy inexpensive snack. It's great for trips packed in plastic bags and presalted or great for the preschooler or kindergarten child to keep at school for snack time. A box of homemade cookies is also easily kept at school for snack time.

This chapter includes substitutes for favorite snacks that you'll no longer be able to buy—popsicles, ice cream cones, ice cream sandwiches, potato chips, pretzels, and so forth. Some of these are easily prepared. Others require more time.

If pizza is dear to your child's heart, don't despair. The pizzas included in this chapter are easily made, delicious, and tomato-free.

Don't exclude from snack time good, nutritious foods like cottage cheese, cheese on crackers, peanut butter on crackers or vegetables, vegetables and dips, fresh fruits, and additive-free nuts (except almonds).

Be sure to avoid the following:

Salicylate fruits
Commercial ice cream cones
Most commercial ice cream

Most commercial crackers, potato chips, pretzels, popcorn, and so forth

Chocolate, at least in the beginning of the diet

Cookies

CAROB COOKIES

Makes 40 cookies

½ cup uncolored butter, softened
¾ cup packed brown sugar
1 egg
1 cup sifted unbleached flour
¼ cup carob powder

½ teaspoon baking powder
¼ teaspoon baking soda
¼ teaspoon salt
1½ teaspoons pure vanilla extract
½ cup chopped walnuts or pecans

Oven 400°

Cream together butter and sugar. Add egg. Mix well. Combine dry ingredients and add to creamed mixture, mixing thoroughly. Add vanilla and nuts and stir well. Drop by teaspoonfuls onto a greased cookie sheet. Bake 8 to 10 minutes.

CAROB OR CHOCOLATE CHIP COOKIES

Makes 3 to 4 dozen cookies

Carob Fudge* makes an excellent substitute for chocolate chips.

½ cup sugar
½ cup packed brown sugar
½ cup uncolored butter, softened
1 egg, slightly beaten
1 teaspoon pure vanilla extract
1 cup unsifted unbleached flour

½ teaspoon baking soda
½ teaspoon salt
¾ cup Carob Fudge* or Baker's German Sweet Chocolate, cut in small pieces
½ cup chopped nuts (optional)

Oven 375°

Cream sugars and butter together. Add egg and vanilla and beat until fluffy. Add dry ingredients and mix well. Fold in chips and nuts. Drop by teaspoonfuls onto ungreased cookie sheet. Bake for 8 to 10 minutes. If cookies spread too much, add a little more flour to remaining batter.

GINGER SNAPS

Makes 3 dozen cookies

¾ cup pure vegetable oil
1 cup packed brown sugar
1 egg
¼ cup molasses
2 cups sifted unbleached
  flour

2 teaspoons baking soda
½ teaspoon salt
½ teaspoon cinnamon
2 teaspoons ginger
¼ cup sugar for dipping

Oven 350°

In a large bowl beat together oil, sugar, egg. Add molasses and mix thoroughly. In a small bowl mix flour, soda, salt, cinnamon, and ginger. Combine contents of both bowls and stir well. Drop by teaspoonfuls into dipping sugar and form into small balls. Place on ungreased cookie sheet 3 inches apart. Oil the bottom of a small glass, dip it in sugar, and flatten each ball. Bake for about 15 minutes.

LEMON AND DATE MACAROONS

Makes 5 to 6 dozen cookies

1 cup uncolored butter,
  softened
1 cup sugar
1 cup packed brown sugar
2 eggs
1 tablespoon pure lemon
  juice
1 teaspoon pure lemon
  extract

¾ cup chopped dates
½ cup chopped nuts
1¼ cups sifted unbleached
  flour
½ teaspoon salt
1 teaspoon baking soda
3 cups rolled oats

Oven 350°

Cream butter and sugars together. Mix in eggs, lemon juice, and extract. Beat thoroughly. Stir in dates and nuts. Add flour, salt, and soda. Mix well. Add oats and mix thoroughly. Measure level tablespoonfuls of dough and put on well-greased cookie sheet. Press mounds flat. Bake for 12 to 15 minutes.

MOLASSES COOKIES

Makes about 6 dozen cookies

1 cup uncolored butter, softened
½ cup sugar
1½ cups light molasses
1 egg, beaten
5 cups sifted unbleached flour

2 teaspoons cinnamon
1 teaspoon nutmeg
1 teaspoon ginger
4 teaspoons baking soda
½ teaspoon salt
½ cup boiling water
Butter Frosting*

Oven 350°

Cream butter and sugar together. Add molasses and egg. Stir in 2 cups flour with spices, soda, and salt. Add boiling water. Mix in remaining flour. Chill for at least 2 hours. Form into balls and place on greased cookie sheets. Press flat with palm of hand. Bake for about 10 minutes. Cool on wire racks. May be frosted with Butter Frosting.*

OATMEAL COOKIES

Makes 6 dozen cookies

2 cups sifted unbleached flour
1¼ cups sugar
1½ teaspoons baking powder
1 teaspoon salt

1 teaspoon cinnamon
3 cups rolled oats
¾ cup chopped nuts
1 cup pure vegetable oil
2 eggs
⅓ cup milk

Oven 350°

Combine first five ingredients. Mix in the rolled oats and nuts. Add oil, eggs, and milk and stir until well blended. Drop from teaspoon onto a greased cookie sheet. Bake for 10 to 12 minutes or until slightly brown.

PEANUT BUTTER COOKIES

Makes 4 dozen cookies

½ cup packed brown sugar
½ cup sugar
½ cup pure vegetable oil
   or uncolored butter,
   softened
1 egg
1 teaspoon pure vanilla
   extract

1 cup peanut butter
1½ cups sifted unbleached
   flour
¼ teaspoon salt
½ teaspoon baking soda
¼ teaspoon baking powder

Oven 375°

In a large bowl combine sugars, oil, egg, and vanilla. Beat until well mixed. Add peanut butter and beat together. In a small bowl mix together flour, salt, soda, and baking powder. Combine contents of both bowls and mix well. Roll dough into small balls about 1 inch in diameter. Place on greased cookie sheet and press flat with a fork. Bake about 15 minutes.

PEAR DROP COOKIES

Makes 3½ dozen cookies

½ cup uncolored butter,
   softened
1 cup packed brown sugar
2 eggs, slightly beaten
1 cup chopped dates
1 cup finely chopped
   canned pears

1 cup rolled oats
½ cup chopped nuts
1¾ cups unbleached flour
½ teaspoon cinnamon
½ teaspoon baking powder
¼ teaspoon salt

Oven 350°

Cream butter and sugar. Add beaten eggs and mix thoroughly. Stir in rest of ingredients. Drop by teaspoonfuls onto a greased cookie sheet. Bake for 15 minutes until lightly browned. Remove from cookie sheet immediately and cool thoroughly before storing.

PINEAPPLE DROP COOKIES

Makes 5 dozen cookies

1 cup uncolored butter, softened
1 cup sugar
1 cup packed brown sugar
2 cups slightly drained unsweetened crushed pineapple
2 eggs, well beaten

1½ teaspoons baking powder
½ teaspoon baking soda
4 cups sifted unbleached flour
1 teaspoon salt
1½ teaspoons pure vanilla extract

Oven 400°

Cream shortening and sugars. Add pineapple and eggs. Mix well. Sift dry ingredients and add to creamed mixture. Blend in vanilla. Drop by spoonfuls onto greased cookie sheet. Bake for 8 to 10 minutes.

QUICK VANILLA COOKIES

Makes 30 cookies

1 egg
½ cup uncolored butter, softened
⅔ cup sugar
1 teaspoon pure vanilla extract

1 cup unbleached flour
½ teaspoon salt
1 teaspoon baking powder

Oven 350°

In a large bowl cream together egg, butter, and sugar. Add vanilla and mix well. Sift together the dry ingredients and gradually add to batter. Drop by teaspoonfuls onto greased cookie sheet. Space about 2 inches apart. Bake for 10 minutes. Remove from cookie sheet and cool on wire rack.

REFRIGERATOR COOKIES

Makes 5 dozen cookies

1 cup pure vegetable oil or uncolored butter, softened
2 cups packed brown sugar
2 eggs
2 teaspoons pure vanilla extract

3½ cups sifted unbleached flour
1 teaspoon baking powder
1 teaspoon salt
1 teaspoon baking soda
1 cup chopped walnuts

Oven 425°

In a large bowl cream oil or butter and brown sugar together. Add eggs one at a time. Stir in vanilla. In another bowl combine dry ingredients. Combine contents of both bowls and then add nuts. Dough will be very firm. On waxed paper shape dough into a roll. Wrap in waxed paper and chill overnight. When ready to bake, cut the dough into little cubes, roll into walnut-size balls, and place on greased cookie sheet. Flatten each ball with a fork. If the edges crumble press together. Bake for about 5 minutes.

SUGAR DROP COOKIES (EGGLESS)

Makes 4 dozen cookies

⅔ cup uncolored butter, softened
¾ cup sugar
1½ teaspoons pure vanilla extract
1 tablespoon milk

1½ teaspoons baking powder
¼ teaspoon salt
1½ cups sifted unbleached flour

Oven 375°

In a large bowl cream together butter, sugar, vanilla, and milk. Sift together dry ingredients and add to batter. Drop by teaspoonfuls onto greased cookie sheet. Bake 10 to 12 minutes. Cool on wire rack.

Crackers

CHEESE WAFERS

Makes 50 crackers

½ cup uncolored butter, softened
2 cups shredded white natural Colby or sharp cheese
1 cup unsifted unbleached flour

1 teaspoon salt
1 teaspoon onion powder (optional)
⅛ teaspoon pepper

Oven 350°

Cream butter and cheese together until well blended. Add remaining ingredients and beat well. Work mixture with your hands and form into two logs about 1½ inches in diameter. Wrap and chill till firm. Using a sharp knife, cut into ⅛-inch slices. Place on ungreased cookie sheet and bake for 12 minutes.

Before baking, crackers may be garnished with nut halves, sesame seeds, herbs, grated Parmesan cheese, and so forth.

COTTAGE CHEESE CRACKERS

Makes about 50
2-inch crackers

1½ cups sifted unbleached
flour
¾ teaspoon salt

½ cup uncolored butter,
softened
½ cup cottage cheese

Oven 450°

In a large bowl mix flour and salt. Add softened butter and cottage cheese. Cut in with pastry blender until well blended. Wrap dough in waxed paper and refrigerate for a least 1 hour.

On a well-floured board roll out dough ⅛ inch thick. Cut out crackers with a 2-inch cookie cutter and place on ungreased baking sheet. Prick each cracker with a fork.

Bake for 12 to 15 minutes until lightly browned. Remove from baking sheet and cool on a rack.

For a more flavorful cracker, grated Parmesan cheese may be sprinkled on crackers before baking.

GRAHAM CRACKERS

Makes 20 2½-inch crackers

½ cup uncolored butter,
softened
½ cup packed brown sugar
¼ cup honey
¼ cup water
2 cups graham or whole
wheat flour

2 tablespoons unbleached
flour
½ teaspoon salt
½ teaspoon cinnamon
1 teaspoon baking powder

Oven 325°

Cream together butter and sugar. Stir in honey and water. Combine all dry ingredients and slowly add to butter mixture. Dough should be stiff. Refrigerate for 30 minutes. Roll out dough on a floured surface until ¼ inch thick. Cut in squares or rounds and place on a well-greased cookie sheet. Bake for about 20 minutes or until bottoms are golden brown.

Others

CARAMEL POPCORN

Makes 3 quarts

¾ cup dark corn syrup
⅓ cup water
1¼ cups sugar
¼ cup uncolored butter

¼ teaspoon salt
½ cup popcorn
¼ cup pure vegetable oil
1 cup salted peanuts

Combine in a saucepan corn syrup, water, sugar, butter, and salt. Bring to a boil over medium heat, stirring constantly. Continue to cook, stirring occasionally, until candy reaches 270° (soft crack stage).

While caramel is cooking, pop corn in oil. Place in a large bowl and mix with peanuts. When caramel is done, quickly pour syrup over popcorn and nuts while stirring briskly until all kernels are covered. Spread on two buttered baking sheets and allow to cool. Break into bite-size pieces and store in a tightly covered container.

CHEESY POPCORN

Makes about 2 quarts

¼ cup pure vegetable oil
⅓ cup popcorn
3 tablespoons uncolored
  butter
2 tablespoons grated
  Parmesan cheese

⅛ teaspoon onion or garlic
  salt (optional)
Salt to taste

Heat oil in 2½-quart saucepan until one corn kernel dropped in pops. Add popcorn. Cover and shake until popcorn stops popping. Remove from heat.

In a small saucepan melt butter. Stir in grated cheese and onion or garlic salt. Pour over hot popcorn. Mix popcorn lightly to distribute butter. Add additional salt to taste.

FROZEN BANANA TREATS

Serves 3

1 4-ounce bar Baker's
  German Sweet
  Chocolate or Carob
  Fudge*

3 medium bananas
½ cup finely chopped nuts

Melt the chocolate or carob fudge (plus milk if needed) in the top of a double boiler over warm water. Drop a banana in the chocolate or carob and carefully spoon over the banana until fully coated. Roll in chopped nuts and place on a waxed-paper-covered pan. Repeat with other bananas. Place in the freezer for several hours until firm.

Leave the bananas whole or cut them into 2-inch pieces, spear with wooden sticks, and serve like popsicles.

GELATIN SNACKS

Makes 25 to 30 snacks

3 envelopes unflavored
  gelatin
½ cup cold water

1 cup sugar
1½ cups unsweetened
  grapefruit juice

In a saucepan sprinkle gelatin over cold water. Place over low heat, stirring constantly until gelatin dissolves. Add sugar and fruit juice and stir over low heat until sugar granules also dissolve.

Pour into a 7×11-inch pan, so that the depth of the liquid is about ½ inch. Chill thoroughly.

Cut out desired shapes with metal cookie cutters, pressing down firmly on the gelatin. Shapes may be decorated with a little icing or left plain. Refrigerate. Use any leftover scraps in other gelatin for color and taste contrasts.

Variations: Replace grapefruit juice with unsweetened pineapple juice, or use cranberry juice cocktail or lemonade, reducing sugar to ¾ cup.

ICE CREAM CONES

Makes 1½ dozen cones

¼ cup uncolored butter
¾ cup confectioners' sugar
2 eggs, beaten
⅛ teaspoon salt
¼ teaspoon pure vanilla
   extract

½ cup sifted unbleached
   flour
2 to 4 tablespoons milk

Melt butter. Set aside until cool. Gradually fold sugar into beaten eggs. Add butter, salt, vanilla, and flour and mix thoroughly. If necessary, thin batter with milk.

Batter may be cooked on a waffle iron preset on medium heat or on a greased griddle. Spread batter thin. Cook 1 to 2 minutes until golden brown on both sides, or drop batter by teaspoonfuls onto a greased and floured cookie sheet, spreading the batter thin. Bake at 300° for 10 to 12 minutes or until golden brown.

After batter has been cooked, remove from waffle iron, griddle, or baking sheet and immediately shape into cones. Secure pointed end of cones with toothpicks until cool. Remove toothpicks. Store unused cones well wrapped in the refrigerator until needed.

ICE CREAM SANDWICHES

Makes 9 squares

2½ cups Graham
   Cracker* crumbs
¾ cup uncolored butter,
   melted

½ cup confectioners' sugar
1½ teaspoons cinnamon
   (optional)
1 quart "safe" ice cream

Mix cracker crumbs with butter, sugar, and cinnamon. Press half the mixture in the bottom of a well-buttered 8×8-inch cake pan. Place in freezer. Chill the remaining crumbs. Soften ice cream. Spread over bottom layer of crumbs until about ½ inch thick. Sprinkle remaining crumbs on top and press them lightly into the soft ice cream. Freeze until firm. To unmold, place pan in hot water. Unmold onto a large piece of foil. Cut immediately into squares. Wrap in foil and return to freezer.

LEMON YOGURT POPS

For yogurt lovers, a good nutritious snack.

Makes 8 to 10 2-ounce pops

16 ounces plain yogurt
3 ounces frozen lemonade concentrate (thawed)
¼ cup confectioners' sugar

Combine yogurt, lemonade, and sugar. Mix well. Pour into small paper cups. Freeze. When almost frozen, place a tongue depressor, plastic spoon, or popsicle stick in the center of each. Freeze until firm. Unmold by placing cups under hot water.

MARSHMALLOW DELIGHTS

Graham Crackers *or brand listed as safe in Appendix B
Marshmallows*
Carob Fudge* or Baker's German Sweet Chocolate

Place graham crackers on a cookie sheet. On half of them place a marshmallow split in half. On the other half place small slices of carob fudge or Baker's German Sweet Chocolate. Heat under the broiler for just a minute or so until marshmallows brown and carob or chocolate begins to melt. Remove immediately. Spread chocolate or carob evenly over graham cracker. Make a "sandwich" by placing one cracker with marshmallow on top of another cracker covered with carob or chocolate. Eat immediately while hot.

POPCORN BALLS

Makes 12 to 15 balls

Follow recipe for Caramel Popcorn,* substituting light corn syrup for dark corn syrup. After spreading popcorn on baking sheet, let cool until you can handle it and form into balls, using your hands. Butter hands to prevent sticking. Wrap each ball in waxed paper and store.

CRANBERRY POPSICLES

Makes 12

¼ cup Simple Sugar Syrup* or
  ½ cup sugar or sweeten to taste
24 ounces cranberry juice cocktail
12 3-ounce paper cups
12 plastic spoons

Dissolve syrup or sugar in cranberry juice. Pour into paper cups. Place a spoon in each cup. Freeze until hard, about 12 hours. To remove popsicle, run hot water over the outside of the cup. Spoon serves as a handle and may be reused.

GRAPEFRUIT OR PINEAPPLE POPSICLES

Makes 12

24 ounces unsweetened
  grapefruit or pineapple
  juice
⅓ cup Simple Sugar Syrup*
  or ⅔ cup sugar or
  sweeten to taste

12 3-ounce paper cups
12 plastic spoons

Prepare as above in Cranberry Popsicles.*

LEMON POPSICLES

Makes 12

½ cup pure lemon juice
2½ cups water
⅓ cup Simple Sugar
  Syrup* or ⅔ cup sugar
  or sweeten to taste

12 3-ounce paper cups
12 plastic spoons

Prepare as above in Cranberry Popsicles.*

PAPAYA POPSICLES

Makes 12

8 ounces commercial (not
   homemade) papaya
   concentrate

2 to 3 cups water
12 3-ounce paper cups
12 plastic spoons

Prepare as above in Cranberry Popsicles.* Sugar is not necessary.

POTATO CHIPS

Baking potatoes
Pure vegetable oil
Salt

Peel as many potatoes as desired. Cut paper-thin rounds from the potatoes using a potato peeler. Drop the slices into cold water. When all the potatoes have been cut up, drain off the water and rinse twice with fresh cold water. Spread out onto paper towels and pat the tops dry with additional towels.

Heat oil (at least 1½ to 2 inches deep) to 370° in a skillet or saucepan. Drop the potato slices into the oil, making sure the slices do not overlap and are not too crowded. Fry for about 30 seconds or until lightly browned. Quickly remove from the oil with a fork or slotted utensil and drain on paper towels. Salt immediately.

These taste exactly like commercial potato chips and do not require a lot of work. Be careful when you are frying them as they will overcook very quickly and will have a burned flavor.

PRETZELS I

Makes about 36 4-inch pretzels

1 package dry yeast or 1
  cake compressed yeast
1 teaspoon sugar
1¼ cups warm water
1 tablespoon salt
3 to 3½ cups unsifted
  unbleached flour

6 cups boiling water
2 tablespoons baking soda
Salt—either regular table
  or coarse salt

Oven 475°

Dissolve yeast and sugar in warm water. Set in a warm place until bubbly. Add salt. Gradually stir in flour until dough is stiff. Place on a floured surface and knead for about 5 minutes or until dough is smooth and elastic. Place in a greased bowl, turning dough once to coat the top. Cover and set in a warm place until double in bulk, about 1 hour. Punch down. Rolling pieces of dough between your hands, form sticks or pretzel shapes. Drop several pretzels at a time into boiling water to which soda has been added. When pretzels float to the top, continue boiling for about 30 to 60 seconds. Drain with a slotted spoon and place on well-greased cookie sheet. Sprinkle well with salt. Bake for about 12 minutes (depending on thickness) or until golden brown. Pretzels will be chewy. May be served with butter and eaten like a bread stick. Store in covered container.

PRETZELS II

Makes 24 pretzels

½ recipe White Bread*
  dough (enough for 1
  loaf) or frozen "safe"
  dough

1 egg yolk
1 tablespoon milk
Salt—either regular table
  or coarse salt

Oven 375°

If using white bread dough, allow to rise once and then firmly punch down. If frozen bread dough is used allow to thaw completely and then work into pretzels.

Cut off walnut-sized pieces of dough and roll on a board with the palms of your hands into thin long round strips about ¼ inch in diameter and 14 to 16 inches long. Twist into pretzel shapes and place on a buttered cookie sheet. Do *not* allow to rise. Combine the egg yolk and milk and brush tops of pretzels with this mixture. Place in the middle of a preheated oven for 15 minutes until golden brown. Remove from oven and immediately brush again with egg yolk mixture and sprinkle with salt. Allow to cool and store.

For a different taste, these pretzels can also be made from Rye Bread* dough.

STUFFED DATES

Slit dates lengthwise. Insert part of a walnut or a whole nut if dates are large. Roll each date in powdered sugar. Keep in covered container in refrigerator.

PIZZA CRUST

Makes 2 12-inch crusts
or 3 9-inch crusts

1 package dry yeast or 1
   cake compressed yeast
1¼ cups warm water
1 teaspoon sugar
3–3½ cups unsifted
   unbleached flour

½ teaspoon salt
1 tablespoon pure
   vegetable oil

Dissolve yeast in warm water. Add sugar. Stir in about half the flour. Add salt. Beat well with an electric mixer for several minutes. Add oil. Work in remaining flour until dough is no longer sticky. On a floured surface, knead dough for 5 to 10 minutes.

Place in a lightly greased bowl, turning dough to coat the top. Cover with a damp cloth and let rise in a warm place until double in bulk. Punch down. Divide dough into desired number of pieces. Roll each piece into a circle. Place on an oiled pizza pan or in cake pans. Turn up the edges. Fill with Pesto or Parsley Pizza filling or Breakfast Fruit Pizza* filling.

Dough may be made earlier in the day. Place in refrigerator where it will slowly rise. If it hasn't doubled in bulk, remove from refrigerator and continue to rise in a warm place. If it rises too much, it may be punched down and allowed to rise again.

PESTO OR PARSLEY PIZZA

Makes 2 12-inch pizzas

1 recipe Pizza Crust*
Pesto* or Parsley Sauce*

½ pound ground beef
8 ounces mozzarella cheese

Oven 350°

Prepare pizza crust. Prepare pesto or parsley sauce. Brown ground beef in a heavy skillet. Drain off excess grease. Add pesto or parsley sauce and heat through. Spread sauce over pizza crust and top with mozzarella cheese. Bake for 20 to 25 minutes until crust is lightly browned.

PIMENTO PIZZA

Makes 1 12-inch pizza

½ recipe Pizza Crust*
½ cup water
1 4-ounce jar pimentos
1 teaspoon sugar
½ teaspoon dried sweet basil
½ teaspoon oregano

1 teaspoon salt
¼ cup pure vegetable oil
1 teaspoon instant minced onion
1 clove garlic
4 ounces mozzarella cheese, shredded

Oven 350°

Prepare pizza crust and place on a greased cookie sheet. Combine rest of ingredients except cheese in a blender and blend until smooth. Pour mixture into a saucepan and bring to a boil. Simmer for 5 minutes. Spread sauce on top of the crust and top with shredded cheese. Bake for 20 to 25 minutes until crust is lightly browned.

CHEESE BALL I

Makes 1 13-ounce ball

1 8-ounce package cream cheese, softened
5 ounce uncolored sharp white cheese, grated

Garlic salt
Dried parsley
Chopped walnuts, pecans, or peanuts

Mix thoroughly cream cheese and sharp cheese with pastry blender or with hands until cheeses are completely blended. Sprinkle garlic salt over the cheese mass and blend it in, using either a pastry blender or your hands. Continue adding garlic salt until desired taste is reached.

Shape cheese into a ball and roll in parsley and chopped nuts until well coated. Refrigerate until serving time. Spread on crackers, bread, or vegetables.

CHEESE BALL II

Makes 1 14-ounce ball

1 8-ounce package cream cheese, softened
2 ounces Roquefort cheese
4 ounces sharp uncolored cheese
1 teaspoon Worcestershire sauce

1 teaspoon instant minced onion
2 tablespoons milk
Parsley flakes
Chopped nuts

Blend cheeses, Worcestershire sauce, onion, and milk together, using your hands. Form into a ball or log and roll in parsley flakes and nuts. Serve with vegetables, crackers, or Potato Chips.*

Beverages

BANANA MILK SHAKE

Makes 2 cups

1 cup milk
1 banana
½ cup "safe" vanilla ice cream

Combine all ingredients in a blender and blend on low speed for 30 to 45 seconds or until smooth. Pour into thermos for lunch box. Shake again before drinking.

CAROB OR CHOCOLATE MILK SHAKE

Makes 1½ cups

1 cup milk
½ cup "safe" vanilla ice cream
2 tablespoons Carob or Chocolate Syrup*

Combine milk and ice cream in a blender. Blend at low speed and pour in syrup while mixing. You can add more ice cream to make a thicker shake. Pour into thermos for lunch box. Shake again before drinking.

EGG NOG

Serves 2

2 cups very cold milk
2 eggs
2 tablespoons sugar or
    honey

½ teaspoon pure vanilla
    extract

Combine ingredients and mix well in a blender or with an electric mixer. Serve at once.

LEMONADE

Makes 1 quart

6 to 8 ounces pure lemon juice
1 to 1½ cups sugar
6 cups cold water

Combine all ingredients. Mix well. Chill.

PEAR NECTAR

Makes 3 cups

1 16-ounce can pears in heavy syrup
1 cup cold water

Place pears and water in blender on high speed until liquefied. Chill thoroughly.

SIMPLE SUGAR SYRUP

1 part sugar
1 equal part water

Combine sugar and water in a heavy saucepan. Stir over medium heat until sugar dissolves. Boil for about 5 minutes without stirring. Refrigerate in a covered container. Use to sweeten fruit juices as desired.

Fruit Fizz Drinks

CRANBERRY FIZZ

Serves 1

6 tablespoons cranberry juice cocktail
1 tablespoon Simple Sugar Syrup*
¼ cup soda water

Combine juice and syrup. Stir in soda water. Add ice cubes.

GRAPEFRUIT FIZZ

Serves 1

¼ cup unsweetened grapefruit juice
1 to 2 tablespoons Simple Sugar Syrup*
4 ounces soda water

Combine juice and syrup. Stir in soda water. Add ice cubes.

LEMON OR LIME FIZZ

Serves 1

2 tablespoons lemon or lime juice
2 to 3 tablespoons Simple Sugar Syrup*
4 ounces soda water

Combine juice and syrup. Stir in soda water. Add ice cubes.

PINEAPPLE FIZZ

Serves 1

¼ cup unsweetened pineapple juice
1 tablespoon Simple Sugar Syrup*
4 ounces soda water

Combine juice and syrup. Stir in soda water. Add ice cubes.

PINEAPPLE-GRAPEFRUIT FIZZ

1 part Pineapple Fizz*
1 equal part Grapefruit Fizz*

Combine and add ice.

13

Candy

Just about all commercial candy is out. It's full of artificial color-ings and flavorings. Don't go overboard in making the candy at home, but if your child has a sweet tooth, surprise him with a treat from time to time as long as he's otherwise eating a well-balanced diet.

You may find a candy thermometer a handy investment if you're going to be making much candy. And there are holidays like Easter and Halloween when candy is traditional. Make the candy in plenty of time so that you'll have time left for preparing and enjoying the holidays. Some candies just can't be duplicated at home—gumdrops, Lifesavers, and so on. However, you'll be able to make delicious substitutes for candy bars that will delight your child and his friends. They may even enjoy helping you, es-pecially making goodies like taffy, which is well suited for a group project. Your child will appreciate a piece of candy tucked in his lunch box. You may wish to include pieces for his friends.

Avoid the following:

> Chocolate, at least in the beginning of the diet
> Colored butter or margarine
> Artificial colorings and flavorings

CAROB FUDGE

Makes 1 pound

¾ cup milk
6 tablespoons sifted carob
  powder
¼ cup uncolored butter
2 cups white or packed
  brown sugar

1 teaspoon pure vanilla
  extract
½ cup chopped walnuts or
  pecans (optional)

Butter sides of heavy saucepan. Combine milk, carob powder, and butter in pan. Bring to a boil, stirring constantly. Add sugar and stir until dissolved. Over medium heat cook without stirring until soft ball stage is reached (234°). Cool to 110° or lukewarm without stirring. Add vanilla and beat until fudge thickens and loses gloss. Fold in nuts. Pour into buttered 9×5-inch loaf pan. Cool. Cut in squares.

CHOCOLATE FUDGE

Makes 2 pounds

3 squares (3 ounces)
  unsweetened chocolate
1⅓ cups milk
3 cups sugar
¼ cup light corn syrup

2 tablespoons uncolored
  butter
1 teaspoon pure vanilla
  extract

Combine chocolate and milk in a medium saucepan. Warm over low heat until the chocolate is completely melted, stirring constantly. Add sugar and corn syrup and bring to a full boil, stirring constantly. Continue to boil, without stirring, until temperature reaches soft ball stage (234°). Remove from heat and add butter and vanilla. Cool mixture until lukewarm. Beat with a spoon until fudge begins to lose its gloss (about 5 minutes). Pour into a buttered 8×8-inch pan and cool until completely set. Cut into squares.

COCONUT CANDY BARS

Makes 20 bite-sized bars

2 cups additive-free coconut
½ cup confectioners' sugar
¼ cup sweetened condensed milk

Combine all ingredients until well mixed. Shape the mixture into small logs about 2 inches long. Chill in refrigerator for 1 hour. Glaze with chocolate or carob.

CREAMY CANDY CENTERS

Makes about 2 dozen balls

1½ cups sugar
¼ teaspoon salt
1 cup pure whipping cream
1 tablespoon water
2 tablespoons uncolored
    butter

¼ cup light corn syrup
1 teaspoon pure vanilla
    extract

Combine all ingredients except vanilla in a saucepan. Bring to a boil, stirring constantly. Continue to boil over medium-low heat, stirring frequently, until the temperature reaches soft ball stage (234°). Immediately remove from heat, add vanilla, and allow to cool until thermometer reads 110°. Quickly stir until candy becomes thick. Drop by teaspoonfuls onto waxed paper. To shape, knead gently and roll until the candy forms a neat ball. Let stand on waxed paper until firm and then coat with chocolate or carob.

LOLLIPOPS

Makes about 40

2 cups sugar
1 cup light corn syrup
½ cup water

1½ teaspoons pure lemon
    extract or pure lime
    extract
Sticks

In a heavy 2-quart saucepan combine sugar, corn syrup, and water. Cook over medium heat, stirring constantly until mixture boils. Continue cooking without stirring until a small amount of mixture dropped into very cold water separates into hard brittle threads (300°). Cool slightly. Add flavoring. Place lollipop sticks 4 inches apart on greased baking sheet or foil. Drop candy syrup from tip of teaspoon over one end of each stick to form a 2-inch disc. If mixture hardens before all lollipops are dropped, stir over low heat until mixture melts.

MARSHMALLOWS

Makes 1½ pounds

2 envelopes unflavored
  gelatin
¾ cup water
1 cup sugar
1 cup light corn syrup

1 egg white
1 teaspoon pure vanilla
  extract
Confectioners' sugar

Soften gelatin in ½ cup cold water. In a heavy saucepan add sugar, corn syrup, and remaining water. Cook until sugar dissolves, stirring constantly. Continue cooking without stirring to soft ball stage (234°). Remove from heat. Add gelatin and stir until dissolved. Cool 10 minutes. Beat egg white until stiff peaks form. Slowly add syrup and vanilla, beating on high speed of electric mixer until mixture forms soft peaks.

Pour onto plain brown paper (a cut-up paper bag is fine) and spread into a rectangle. Let stand overnight. Dust top with confectioners' sugar. Turn over onto waxed paper. Moisten brown paper with a sponge or cloth until paper is easily peeled away from candy. Using kitchen shears, cut into pieces and roll edges in confectioners' sugar.

CAROB OR CHOCOLATE MARSHMALLOWS

Using above recipe, add 1 to 2 tablespoons carob powder or cocoa when sugar, corn syrup, and water are combined.

NUTTY CARAMELS

Makes 1½ pounds

½ cup uncolored butter
1¼ cups packed brown
 sugar
⅛ teaspoon salt
½ cup light corn syrup
1 cup sweetened condensed
 milk

1 teaspoon pure vanilla
 extract
½ cup chopped nuts
 (optional)

Melt butter in a heavy saucepan. Add sugar, salt, and corn syrup. Mix well. Add milk, stirring constantly. Cook over medium heat to firm ball stage (245°), about 15 minutes, stirring constantly. Remove from heat. Add vanilla and nuts. Mix well. Pour into buttered 8×8- or 9×9-inch pan. Cool thoroughly. Using kitchen shears, cut into squares.

This may be used for candy bars by cutting into 1×3-inch pieces and coating with chocolate or carob.

CAROB CARAMELS

Add ¼ cup carob powder before stirring in milk.

PEANUT BRITTLE

Makes 2 pounds

1½ cups light corn syrup
1½ cups sugar
¾ cup water
½ cup uncolored butter
2 cups salted additive-free
 peanuts

1 teaspoon baking soda
1 teaspoon pure vanilla
 extract

In a medium saucepan combine corn syrup, sugar, and water. Cook over medium heat, stirring constantly, until boiling. Blend in butter and cook, stirring frequently, until the temperature reaches

280°. Add peanuts and continue to boil to 305° (hard crack stage), stirring constantly. Remove from heat and stir in baking soda and vanilla until well mixed. Pour onto buttered cookie sheets. When completely cool, loosen and crack into bite-size pieces.

PEANUT BUTTER FUDGE

Makes about 2½ pounds

2 cups sugar
⅓ cup light corn syrup
⅔ cup evaporated milk
¼ teaspoon salt
2 tablespoons uncolored butter
1 teaspoon pure vanilla extract

½ cup additive-free (may contain salt) smooth or crunchy peanut butter
1½ cups chopped walnuts or pecans (optional)

Combine sugar, corn syrup, milk, and salt in a heavy saucepan. Cook over medium heat to a soft ball stage (234°). Remove from heat. Add butter, vanilla, and peanut butter, and beat with an electric mixer until fudge begins to stiffen. Fold in nuts if desired. Turn into buttered pan. Cool. Cut into pieces.

PEANUT CLUSTERS

Makes 24

4 ounces Baker's German Sweet Chocolate
1 to 1½ cups salted additive-free peanuts

Melt chocolate in top of double boiler. Stir in peanuts. Drop by teaspoonfuls onto waxed paper. Allow to harden.

TAFFY

Makes 1 pound

1¼ cups light corn syrup
1 cup water
2¼ cups sugar
½ teaspoon salt

2 teaspoons pure vanilla
extract
1 tablespoon uncolored
butter

Combine corn syrup, water, sugar, and salt in a medium saucepan and bring to a boil, constantly. Discontinue stirring and continue to cook until the temperature reaches 254° (hard ball stage). Remove from heat and stir in vanilla and butter thoroughly. Pour onto a buttered cookie sheet. When cool enough to handle, butter hands and twist and pull taffy until it becomes creamy white. Pull into long strips and twist. Cut into 1-inch pieces with scissors and wrap in squares of waxed paper.

VANILLA FUDGE

Makes 1 pound

2 cups sugar
⅔ cup milk, light cream, or
evaporated milk
⅓ cup uncolored butter

1 tablespoon pure vanilla
extract
½ cup chopped walnuts or
pecans (optional)

Butter sides of heavy saucepan. Combine sugar, milk, and butter in saucepan over medium heat. Stir until sugar dissolves and mixture comes to a boil. Let boil over medium heat until soft ball stage (234°) is reached. Remove from heat. Let stand until temperature reaches 110° or bottom of pan is comfortably warm. Add vanilla. Beat until creamy and thickened. Stir in nuts. Pour into well-greased 8-inch-square pan. When firm, cut into pieces.

CHOCOLATE COATING FOR CANDIES

1 to 2 pounds Baker's German Sweet Chocolate
Assorted candy centers

Break the chocolate into small chunks and place in the top of a double boiler. Pour hot, not boiling, water into the bottom of the pan. Place on the stove and turn on to a *very* low heat, just enough to keep the water warm. Do not let the water boil. Stir the chocolate until it is completely melted. Drop a piece of candy into the chocolate and turn it over with a fork until it is coated on all sides. A fondue fork, or any two-tined fork, works well. Lift the candy out of the chocolate with the fork and place on a piece of waxed paper. Allow the candy to set for several hours and then store for future use.

CAROB COATING FOR CANDIES

To coat candy centers with carob use plain carob candy bars, which can be found in health food stores and some grocery stores now. Melt them in the top of a double boiler and dip centers as you would for Chocolate Coating for Candies.* Or prepare Carob Fudge* without nuts. To use for dipping, place fudge in top of double boiler and melt over hot water. Several drops of milk may be needed to thin fudge just a little.

14

Holiday and Birthday Suggestions

For the hyperactive child parties and holidays are particularly difficult times. The excitement of these special occasions plus a high intake of party-type foods, which are usually artificially colored and flavored often cause tears, heartbreak, and chaos. But take heart! With a little forethought and planning you can have delicious holiday meals and party menus that delight everyone.

Your positive attitude about the diet will make these occasions easier for your child and, therefore, for the whole family. Don't make a great fuss about having to do extra cooking. Cut menus down to what you can easily handle. A great variety is not necessarily needed but make each item you cook the best and serve it attractively. Holidays will be more enjoyable and relaxed for everyone as your hyperactive child calms down.

The traditional holidays involving family-type dinners should be relatively simple since they usually call for good home-cooked foods easily adapted to the limits of the diet. For example, the traditional Thanksgiving menu at our house calls for

Turkey with Stuffing*
Cranberry Jelly*
Mashed Potatoes with Homemade Gravy
Sweet Potatoes
Buttered Peas and/or Green Beans
No-Knead White Refrigerator Rolls* with Uncolored Butter
Pumpkin Pie* with Whipped Cream or Whipped Topping*

This dinner should not present a problem as far as the diet is concerned. Much of this menu you probably have been cooking for years. Of course, most instant potatoes, packaged stuffings, or prepared gravies cannot be used. These are not major problems and any extra effort can be minimized by additional preparation beforehand.

The rolls, cranberry jelly, and pie all can be made the day before and therefore leave your day to devote mainly to the turkey. Remember you cannot use a self-basting turkey so allow yourself extra time.

For Christmas dinner you could use the following menu:

> Beef Roast with Homemade Gravy
> Browned Potatoes
> Lima Beans with Mushrooms*
> Fruit Salad with Fruit Salad Dressing*
> Corn Muffins*
> Vanilla Ice Cream* with Snowball Cupcakes*

The only items that may need special attention are the ice cream, corn muffins, and the snowball cupcakes.

Prepared corn muffin mixes may have to be avoided (check the labels) and the ice cream must be either a commercial natural product or homemade. To make the snowball cupcakes use the Cupcakes* recipe in Chapter 10 and bake in greased and lightly floured muffin pans without using paper liners. When the cakes are cooled, round off any edges with a sharp knife and completely ice all sides. Gently roll or pat flaked additive-free coconut on the top and sides. Top with a small red birthday candle and serve.

At our house Christmas cookies are always a special treat. We use them for gifts, snacks, and treats when guests drop in. You probably will find that most cookie recipes you now use are basically all right with few or no changes. Use chopped dates where raisins are called for, pecans or walnuts for almonds. A mixture of cinnamon and nutmeg will substitute nicely for cloves, and pineapple or pears replace most other fruits in baked goods. Use uncolored butter and unbleached flour. Don't give up your favorite recipe because it calls for an item on the forbidden list. You can usually find a suitable substitute.

On Valentine's Day you can add your own special touch. Make

a cake using heart-shaped pans and frost using an icing colored pink with cranberry juice. If heart-shaped pans are not available use one 8-inch round layer pan and one 8-inch-square pan to make the cake. Cut the round layer in half and place the cut edges against two adjacent sides of the square cake to form a heart.

Since the diet will not allow you to rely on bakery cakes and pastries and will entail more baking for holidays and parties, you might consider investing in special pans and molds that will give you more flexibility. Many of these items are available rather inexpensively at your local department store or through several mail order houses.

For a Valentine party at school, volunteer to make the treats for the class so you can regulate what your child has to eat. Make his favorite cookies and top with icing tinted pink with cranberry juice cocktail. For a drink bring Cranberry Fizz* and serve with Valentine napkins and cups.

An easy Easter dinner menu might include the following:

> Leg of Lamb
> Scalloped Potatoes*
> Asparagus and Egg Casserole*
> Molded Vegetable Salad*
> Pineapple Muffins*
> Egg-shaped Coconut Cake

An old canned ham container makes a great pan for an egg-shaped cake. Be sure, however, that the pan is not coated with plastic and is entirely metal. Bake the cake in the ham container, ice and coat with additive-free coconut. Place fresh flowers on top for a touch of spring.

The candy associated with Easter will likely have to be homemade. If your child is old enough, he may even enjoy helping you make his favorites. Peanut Clusters,* Carob Caramels,* Marshmallows,* Coconut Candy Bars,* and Creamy Candy Centers* are some that could be prepared to fill an Easter basket. The creamy candy centers can be molded into large and small egg shapes and then coated with carob, chocolate, or a colored icing. Add piping of different colored icings to decorate. Wrapping the individual pieces of candy in colorful papers such as aluminum foil or foil gift wrapping paper gives a festive look. Commercial fancy carob Easter eggs are beginning to appear in health food stores. Read labels carefully.

Hard-boiled eggs can be easily colored with the natural food dyes listed in Chapter 2 or decorated with marking pens in bright colors. Plastic eggs that open can be filled with coins or small toys. These are found in novelty stores and can be painted with flowers, designs, or even the child's name.

Again, by having a party at your house, you can regulate what your child eats. An Easter egg hunt can be arranged using a combination of regular hard-boiled eggs colored with safe natural dyes and plastic eggs filled with homemade candies, coins, toys, etc. Follow the hunt with cookies or cupcakes for the guests and a fruit punch.

A yearly event at our house is decorating blown egg shells and hanging them on an egg tree. Bring in a sturdy branch from outside and anchor it in a large flower pot filled with sand. Glue ribbon loops to the tops of the blown eggs for hanging. We save these eggs from year to year and always add a few new ones. If there is a budding artist in your house, some very fancy eggs can be done, but usually we all create our own designs.

The Fourth of July is a perfect time for a summer get-together and outdoor party. The dress is casual and the food should be typical picnic fare.

> Barbecued Chicken*
> Baked Potatoes on the Grill
> Roast Corn on the Cob
> Red, White, and Blue Holiday Salad*
> Baked Beans*
> Watermelon

The barbecued chicken should be basted with a tomato-less-type sauce. Cook the chicken entirely on the grill. Or bake it covered in your kitchen oven for 45 minutes, then cook another 15 to 20 minutes outside on the grill until it is completely done and has that good smoky taste.

Both the baked potatoes and corn on the cob can be done on the grill. Simply grease and wrap potatoes in aluminum foil and cook over the coals for 1 hour. Corn on the cob can be cooked right in the husk on the grill. Soak corn several hours in cold water. When ready to grill, drain and place over hot coals, turning frequently for 20 to 25 minutes or until done.

The baked beans and red, white, and blue holiday salad can be made ahead of time. An ice cold watermelon tops off an easy, delicious dinner.

You have several options when holiday dinners are at places other than your home. Many relatives and friends will co-operate completely when you explain the diet and its merits. If you feel this is possible, by all means try it. They can at least tell you their planned menu so that any "unsafe" foods can be avoided. You might offer to bring one or more items you know your child enjoys and are safe.

You also have the option of completely forgetting the diet for the day. This does have obvious consequences and you must weigh the pros and cons carefully. As the diet becomes more familiar and you discover how your child reacts when he has a particular forbidden food you can then decide how serious the effects may be. If only a mild reaction is the result, it may be worth the splurge, but if a violent upset results you must decide if it is worth it. Don't forget that the next day you must return to the diet. Explain this to your child beforehand so he understands the circumstances.

The trick or treats at Halloween are not easily solved. You may decide to let your child forget the diet on this occasion. Of course, you have control over the candy that is given out at your home but treats from others are usually loaded with additives. If your neighbors understand and sympathize with your problem, they may co-operate by making a special treat for your trick-or-treater. This may work for a small child but practically speaking an older one may want to join in the fun.

Once your child realizes the benefits of the diet he may co-operate in these situations. Maybe he can go trick or treating with the others and give what he has collected to a sick child who could not go out that night. Donating his goodies to an orphanage or a needy family may be in order. Trick or treating for UNICEF could be an answer. Talk it over with your child and do what he feels comfortable with. Make an extra treat for him at home so he can have something special to eat as a reward for his co-operation.

Staying home to give out the treats makes children feel grown-up and may be just the solution. Our neighbors dress in scary costumes themselves to give out the treats and join in the fun. Another Halloween idea is taking pictures of trick-or-treaters as they visit your house and giving the snapshots to the children. An older child can be the photographer and therefore feel very much a part of the evening.

Popcorn balls, doughnuts, homemade candy bars, or taffy are always welcome treats. You will become a real hit at Halloween because of these special goodies, so make plenty.

Birthday Parties

To children birthdays are very important events and should be special. Hyperactive children, particularly preschoolers, usually cannot cope with a large birthday party. Tears, fights, temper tantrums, and overexcitement are extremely common. For a very young child a family celebration is usually all that is necessary. There are other ways to make the day special—a movie, ball game, circus, ice skating, and so on. Your child may wish to ask one or two friends too and afterward invite them home for homemade ice cream and cake. Selecting the dinner menu for the family celebration also makes the day extra special.

If your child has calmed down on the diet or has his heart set on a party, limit the number of guests to what you can accommodate and enlist extra help if necessary. Food for the party need not be fancy since children generally don't like to try new or exotic things away from home.

If you have been purchasing all the party foods in the past, of course, you now must prepare some yourself. There are several additive-free ice creams on the market that you can serve (see list in Appendix B). If you do not have access to one of these or prefer to make your child's favorite for his birthday, do so several days in advance of the party.

Sometimes the ice cream making can be part of the party entertainment. Children are fascinated by an ice cream freezer and love to join in making their own. If you don't own a freezer, maybe a good neighbor will loan you one for the party.

A hand-crank unit can keep the children busy with each taking a turn at cranking or adding ice. An electric unit is easier to use and still is exciting to watch. Follow the recipes (using "safe" ingredients) and instructions that come with the freezer and you should not go wrong even on the first try. Remember that the freezer requires constant watching and with smaller children an adult must supervise.

Ice cream served right from the crank freezer will be soft and creamy. If you want to harden it, put it in your refrigerator freezer for a time while the children are playing games or opening presents at the party. Either way you can be sure the kids will love it.

Cakes are the most important treat and a must at every birthday party. The traditional cake, of course, is one with "Happy Birthday" written on top with colored icing and candles counting out the child's age. If this is the favorite at your house, you should have no trouble duplicating this from an acceptable diet recipe that will make the birthday child quite happy.

When a different cake decoration is requested there are lots of items and ideas available. Choosing a hobby or pastime as a theme for your cake and party is always a good place to start. Shop around for miniature trains, baseball caps, bicycles, dolls, airplanes, or dancers to decorate the top of the cake. Favorite fairy tales or stories about circuses, zoos, or animals also can be used as a theme. For his fifth birthday, Jack was thrilled by a cake decorated with small finger puppets of his favorite Sesame Street characters.

Plastic, metal, or wooden items should be placed on the cake immediately before serving and removed quickly. Dyes and paints on these products could be transmitted to the icing.

Fresh flowers placed around the base and on top of a cake are lovely and add a pretty, feminine touch. This works well for the older girl or for Mom's birthday.

The Gelatin Snacks* in Chapter 12 can be made into cake decorations too. Pour the gelatin mixture into a shallow pan so that it is ⅛ inch deep. Chill until thoroughly set and cut with cookie cutters into animals, stars, or other interesting shapes. Lay these on the top of an iced cake for a different look.

Another idea for a decorative cake is cutting an ordinary 13×9-inch cake into numbers representing the age of the birthday child. Use the following chart to cut the cake and frost the top and

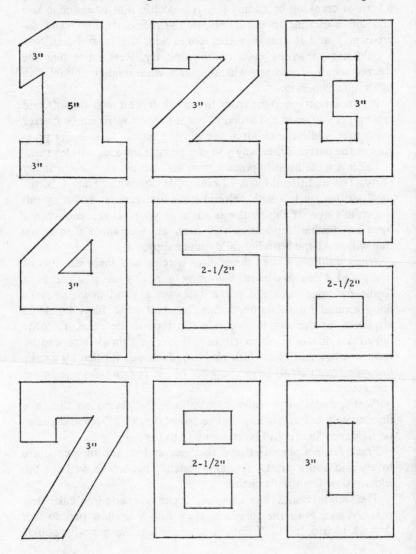

sides. Trim the edges with carob or colored piping and add candles.

Following are several birthday party suggestions to help you get started. There are party menus, themes, centerpieces, favors, cakes, and decoration ideas that can be used as they are or you can modify them as you wish.

Ship Ahoy Party

MENU

Ship-shape Cake
Ice Cream
Cranberry Fizz*

Centerpiece: Use a model sailing ship sitting on a mirror to represent water.

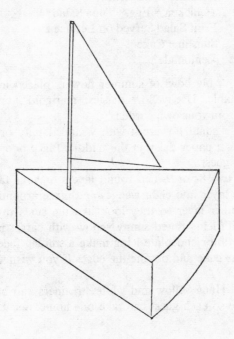

Favors: Wrap small toy boats as gifts or use boats folded from paper and filled with salted nuts.

Cake: Bake two 8- or 9-inch cake layers of yellow cake or carob cake. Cut each single layer into six wedge-shaped pieces. Frost the tops and all sides of each piece. Make sails for each "ship" out of straws and construction paper. Stick sails on each piece of cake and serve with scoops of ice cream of your favorite flavor and cranberry fizz.

Decorations: Sailor hats for each child can be made from paper or purchased inexpensively. Paper plates, napkins, and cups in red, white, and blue with a bunch of balloons hanging from the ceiling should be all you need.

Summer Sunshine Party

MENU

Assorted Sandwiches
(Chicken,* Egg,* Tuna Salad*)
Fruit Salad Served on Lettuce Leaf
Sunshine Cake*
Lemonade*

Centerpiece: A big bowl of summer flowers placed in the middle of the table. Use yellow daisies, marigolds, or a bouquet picked from your own garden.

Favors: Fill a small flowerpot with wrapped taffy or salted nuts and stick a paper daisy in the middle. Place one on the table for each guest.

Cake: Bake two 8- or 9-inch round layers of your favorite cake. Cut one layer into eight wedges and place around the outside of the other layer so they look like the sun's rays. Frost all sides with icing tinted sunny yellow with carrot juice. With a little carob or chocolate icing make a smiling face in the center of the cake and outline the edges if you wish. Add candles and serve.

Decorations: Hang yellow and white streamers and balloons over the table so each guest can take one home. Set the table with bright yellow paper plates and napkins on a light green table-cloth.

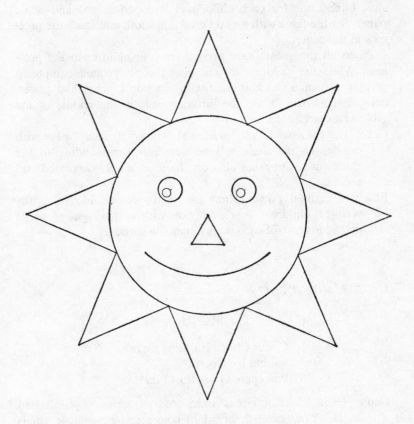

Picnic Party

MENU

Fried Chicken*
Potato Chips*
Celery and Carrot Sticks
Pineapple Fizz*
Birthday Cake or Cupcakes*

Take your party guests to a nearby park or, if you have the facilities, your own back yard. Bring the food packed in individual shoe boxes, one for each child, and wrapped in red and white paper. Set the table with a checkered tablecloth and stack the presents in the center.

When all the guests have arrived let your child open the presents. While the children are enjoying the playground equipment or playing games, set the table with the box lunches and plates, cups, and napkins. Place the birthday cake in the middle of the table as a centerpiece.

Cake: The cake can be the traditional "Happy Birthday" cake with candles or the shape of the numeral corresponding to the child's age. Cupcakes also can be individually decorated and served.

Favors: A small potted plant for each guest is intriguing for younger children. A clever pot with a package of seeds tucked inside will encourage a budding gardener.

Circus Clown Party

MENU

Circus Clown Birthday Cake*
Vanilla Ice Cream*
Pineapple-Grapefruit Fizz*

Centerpiece: Make a circus train from a series of cardboard boxes. Spray paint them bright colors and put plastic circus animals in each car.

Favors: Have cone-shaped hats for each child to wear and a small wrapped toy at each place. Yo-yos, jacks, jump ropes, balls, card games, or puzzle books are good choices.

Cake: Make a clown cake using one 8-inch-round and one 8-inch-square layer. Cut and assemble as indicated below. Frost the cake using either colored icings or all white icing and use small bits of tinted icing to outline and add features. To serve the ice cream, homemade cones may be placed on top of a scoop of ice cream to form a clown's hat. Make a face on the ice cream with blueberries for eyes and cranberries for a mouth.

Decorations: Hang crepe paper streamers in a bunch from the ceiling with the end of each streamer leading to the gift-wrapped favor at each place. Use paper products in a circus design for the table.

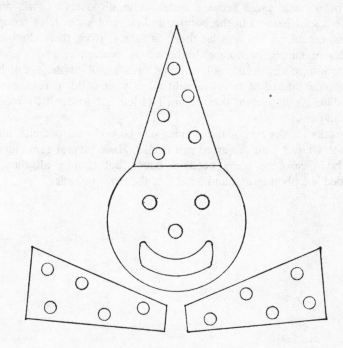

Teen-age Dinner Party

MENU

Hamburgers on Sandwich Buns* with all the trimmings
Potato Salad*
Vegetable Relish tray with Zippy Curry Dip*
Banana Splits
"Safe" Soft Drinks (See Appendix B)

Teen-agers like relaxed and informal parties and usually generate their own fun. Since hamburgers are a teen-age must they are certain to be a hit. Serve the dinner buffet style and let each guest put on his own trimmings. Make sure you fix plenty.

Potato salad and a relish tray of green onions, radishes, olives, celery, and carrot sticks complete the dinner.

For dessert, again serve a buffet. Use disposable bowls and place a split banana in the bottom and sides of each. Dish scoops of ice cream on top and let the kids take it from there. Provide dishes of carob, chocolate, butterscotch, pineapple, and marshmallow toppings, nuts, and whipped cream. All of these can be homemade ahead of time and will allow your child to remain on the diet. It's important that he not feel left out so don't fix foods he can't eat.

Snacks for the rest of the evening can be popcorn, peanuts, and Potato Chips* with the usual soft drinks. Have several game ideas ready in case the party needs a boost, but usually all that is needed is a phonograph and a stack of the latest records.

APPENDIX A: The Diet

We recommend starting the diet by eliminating *all* foods *not permitted* in the three groups listed below. However, at the start, you may prefer to remove only foods not permitted in Group One. If you are not totally successful or achieve no changes or feel more progress is possible, eliminate also the prohibited foods in Group Two. Again, if your child's behavior has not improved as much as you hoped, then eliminate foods prohibited in all three groups.

Group One: Artificial Colorings and Flavorings

FOODS NOT PERMITTED

—Eliminate any food to which your particular child reacts negatively.
—Chocolate seems to be an extremely common example so you should eliminate it at the start of the diet. Carob bean products (may be purchased in health food stores and elsewhere) may be used as a chocolate substitute as noted in many of our recipes.
—Foods containing artificial colorings and flavorings are *not* permitted. Read labels on *all* foods you buy for such information. Some cheeses, butter, and ice cream are not required by law to list a coloring additive, so you may have to check with the manufacturer.
—The following is a list of popular foods and other substances usually containing artificial colorings and flavorings:

Most commercial ice cream, sherbet, ices, gelatins, puddings, etc.
Flavored yogurt

Frozen fish fillets or sticks that are dyed or flavored
Hams, bacon
Luncheon meats, hot dogs,

Chocolate milk
Margarine
Most butters
Many cheeses
Prepared gravies
Mustard, mayonnaise
Soy sauce, if colored or flavored
Artificial vanilla (vanillin)
    flavoring
Gum
Most commercial candies
Some bakery goods
Cake mixes, pudding mixes,
    gelatin mixes, prepared
    piecrusts, etc.
All barbecued poultry, all stuffed
    poultry, all self-basting
    turkeys

chipped beef, corned beef,
    sausage, etc.
Some commercial soups and
    broths
Many prepared pickles are
    artificially colored
Kool-Aid and other similar
    products
Soda pop
Diet drinks and supplements
Frozen limeade often contains
    artificial coloring
Toothpaste—salt and baking soda
    may be used as a substitute
Cough drops, Lifesavers
Mouthwash, throat lozenges
Vitamin pills, medications—ask
    your doctor

FOODS PERMITTED

Uncolored butter, uncolored
    cheeses (cheese may have
    other additives)
Homemade ice cream or
    completely natural ice cream
Plain yogurt
White milk
Honey
Pure vanilla, lemon, or lime
    extracts
Unflavored gelatin
Homemade candy with no
    artificial colorings or
    flavoring
Homemade mustard, mayonnaise

Cereals without artificial colorings
    and flavorings and without
    raisins (prohibited in Group
    Two)
Distilled white vinegar
7-Up
Sprite
Teem
Baking soda and salt for
    toothpaste
Adult white Tylenol tablets or
    similar-type compounds (no
    aspirin) for pain or fever—
    check with your doctor for
    use and dosage

Group Two:

FOODS NOT PERMITTED

—Fruits and vegetables containing natural salicylates are not permitted:

Apples
Almonds
Apricots
Blackberries
Boysenberries
Cherries
Cloves, allspice
Cucumbers and cucumber pickles, relish
Currants
Gooseberries
Grapes
Mint flavors
Nectarines
Oil of wintergreen
Oranges

Peaches
Plums, prunes
Raisins
Raspberries
Strawberries
Cider and cider vinegar, wine and wine vinegar
Gin and all distilled drinks, beer
Jellies, jams made from any fruits on this list and/or artificially colored or flavored
All tea
Tomatoes and all tomato products —catsup, chili sauce, steak sauces, tomato paste, etc.

FOODS PERMITTED

Avocados
Bananas
Blueberries
Cranberries, cranberry juice
Dates
Grapefruit, grapefruit juice
Guava, guava nectar
Lemons, homemade lemonade, pure lemon juice
Limes, homemade limeade, pure lime juice

Nuts other than almonds
Pears
Pineapple, pineapple juice
Rhubarb
All vegetables except tomatoes and cucumbers as noted above
Non-cucumber pickles are okay but many commercial brands contain artificial coloring and cannot be used

Group Three:

FOODS NOT PERMITTED

—Omit other additives, in particular BHA and BHT. Avoid bleached white flour which contains bleaching and maturing agents.
   —BHA (butylated hydroxyanisole) and BHT (butylated hydroxytoluene) are preservatives and must be listed on labels. BHA and BHT are commonly found in shortenings, oils, potato chips, bakery products, dry yeast, etc.

FOODS PERMITTED

—Unbleached, naturally matured flour.
—Homemade breads made from this "safe" flour; also homemade cookies, crackers, buns, etc.
—Pure vegetable oils with no preservatives may be purchased in some grocery stores or health food stores.
—Yeast cakes found in refrigeration case of grocery store or packages of dry yeast with no BHA or BHT.

APPENDIX B: Safe Brands

The following brands are "safe" to use as far as we have been able to determine. However, manufacturers may change their ingredients or processing from time to time. If you have any doubts, check with the companies. No doubt there are many other equally "safe" brands to be found in your area. Check labels carefully and contact manufacturers as needed.

Dairy Products

Uncolored Butter	Land O' Lakes *Unsalted* Sweet Butter
Uncolored, Unbleached Cheese	County Line—Colby Sharpy, Old World, Swiss
	Kraft white cheeses such as Parmesan, Brick, Munster, Swiss, Mozzarella, Monterey Jack
	Kraft yellow cheeses are dyed with *natural vegetable* dyes
	Brie, Camembert, Roquefort, and Limburger are cheeses free of colorings and preservatives
	No colorings may be added to Parmesan cheese although it may contain preservatives
Ice Cream	Breyer's Ice Creams
	Lady Borden Ice Creams
	Meadow Gold Old Fashioned Recipe

Flours and Breads

Unbleached, Naturally Matured Flours	Harrington's Hodgson Mill
	Pillsbury Unbleached White
	Elam's
	El Molino
Frozen Bread Dough	Rhodes Frozen White or Whole Wheat Bread, Rolls. (Rhodes offers a great little cookbook filled with ideas based on their frozen dough.)

	Catherine Clark's Brownberry Ovens Home Baking Dough
Bread Mixes	Elam's Bread Mixes
	Catherine Clark's Brownberry Oven Mixes
	Flako Corn Muffin Mix
	Aunt Jemima Easy Corn Bread Mix, Self-Rising Corn Meal Mix
Baked Loaves	Catherine Clark's Brownberry Oven White, Corn, Oatmeal, Natural Wheat
	Pepperidge Farm (contains calcium propionate to retard spoilage) English Muffins, Wheat Bread, Whole Wheat Rolls

Chocolate and Carob

Carob Powder	El Molino Cara Coa Carob Powder
Chocolate	Hershey's Baking Chocolate, Unsweetened
	Baker's Unsweetened Chocolate
	Baker's German Sweet Chocolate

Snacks

Crackers and Cookies	Nabisco Premium Saltines
	Nabisco Graham Crackers (in the red box)
	Nabisco Cinnamon Treats
	Nabisco Triscuits (have BHA, BHT)
	Fritos (have BHA, BHT)
	Venus Wheat Wafers
	Ralston Purina Original Rye Crisp
	Flavor Tree Onion, Cheddar, and Sesame Crackers
	Pepperidge Farm Cookies
	Pepperidge Farm Goldfish (Pretzel or Lightly Salted)
	Nature Valley Honey 'n Oats Granola Bars
Candy	Cracker Jack
	Reese's Peanut Butter Cups (contain chocolate)
	Golden Harvest Pure Carob Swirls
	Joan's Natural Candies
	Cara Coa Candy Bar
Potato Chips, Pretzels	Charles Chips
	Country Oven Potato Chips
	Crane Corn Chips
	Wege Hard Pretzels

Beverages

Soda Pop   7-Up, Sprite, Teem (contain no artificial
                        colors or flavors, do contain other
                        additives)

Carob, Cocoa   Cara Coa Carob Drink
                        Swiss-Miss Instant Cocoa Mix

Cereals

Cold   Post Grape Nuts
                        Quaker Puffed Rice or Wheat
                        Quaker 100% Natural Cereal
                        Pet Incorporated Heartland Natural Cereal
                          (Plain)
                        Golden Harvest Puffed Wheat
                        Golden Harvest Corn Flakes
                        Van Brode Special Corn Flakes
                        Nature Valley Granola

Hot   Quaker Old Fashioned Oats, Quick Quaker
                          Oats, Cream of Wheat (5 min.)
                        Wheatena

Miscellaneous Items

Yeast   Red Star Dry Yeast
                        Fleischmann's Compressed Yeast Cakes

Coconut   Bakers Southern Style Coconut, Bakers
                          Angel Flake

Mayonnaise   Kraft Real Mayonnaise, Miracle Whip
                          Salad Dressing
                        Hunza
                        Hain
                        Hollywood

Lemon Juice   Minute Maid 100% Pure Lemon Juice
                          (in freezer case)

Extracts   McCormick's Pure Vanilla Extract,
                          Pure Lemon Extract

Luncheon Meats   Health Maid Franks and Bologna (frozen)

Cranberry Jelly   Ocean Spray

APPENDIX C: Evaluating the Results of the Diet

Grading System: Number of points and meaning of each grade.

MEANING		GRADE	POINT VALUE
Beautiful, happy time, little or no hyper-activity, very reasonable		A	11
	A—	10	
	B+	9	
Better than usual, a noticeable improvement	B	8	
	B—	7	
	C+	6	
An average day with your child before starting the diet	C	5	
	C—	4	
	D+	3	
A lousy day, child hyper and/or fussy, whiny, everyone tense, unhappy	D	2	
	D—	1	
Total chaos, everyone unhappy, child completely out of control, unreachable	F	0	

If you see your child mornings, afternoons, and evenings, grade each time period and keep a record of the grades. At the end of the day, add up the total points and put the result on the graph paper provided on the next page. You are making progress when the graph begins to climb above the average line (15 points a day if you're grading your child three times a day).

If your child is in school and you observe him only in the afternoons and evenings, then grade the portions of the day you see him and graph the results.

If you can see that he's making progress, but suddenly the graph turns downward, check back in your daily food diary and note what changes you made in his diet when your child begain to go downhill.

Four Week Evaluation Graph

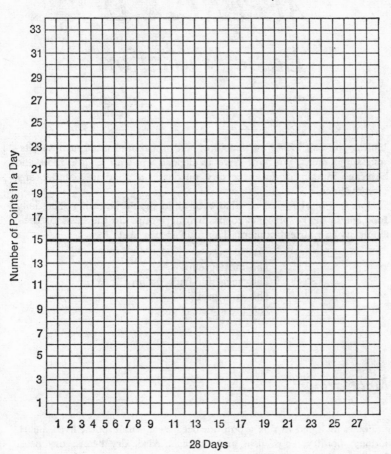

APPENDIX D:
Basic Nutrition

Unless you can locate an uncolored and unflavored multipurpose vitamin supplement, you will have to depend on your child's food and beverage intake for his necessary nutrients, a good idea under any circumstance.

Here is a brief review of what your child should be eating. The daily food guide below presents foods in four groups on the basis of their similarity in nutrient content. The four groups are:

> The meat group
> The vegetable-fruit group
> The milk group
> The bread-cereal group

Meat Group

Foods included in this group are beef, veal, lamb, pork, liver, heart, kidney, poultry, eggs, fish, and shellfish. Also, dry beans, dry peas, lentils, nuts, peanuts, and peanut butter.

Amounts recommended: Choose two or more servings per day. Count as a serving: 2 to 3 ounces lean, boneless cooked meat, poultry, or fish, two eggs, 1 cup cooked dry beans, dry peas, or lentils, or ¼ cup peanut butter.

Vegetable-Fruit Group

Foods included in this group are all vegetables and fruits. Particularly important are those that are valuable as sources of vitamin C and vitamin A.

Good sources of vitamin C but without salicylates are grapefruit, grapefruit juice, cantaloupe, guava, mango, papaya, broccoli, Brussels sprouts, green pepper, sweet red pepper, pineapple juice (if fortified with ascorbic acid), and cranberry juice (if fortified with ascorbic acid).

Fair sources of vitamin C include honeydew melon, lemons, lemonade, watermelon, asparagus tips, raw cabbage, collards, garden cress, kale, mustard greens, potatoes and sweet potatoes cooked in the jacket, spinach and turnip greens.

Good sources of vitamin A are dark green and deep yellow vegetables and a few fruits—broccoli, cantaloupe, carrots, chard, collards, cress, kale, mango, pumpkin, spinach, sweet potatoes, turnip greens and other dark green leafy vegetables, and winter squash.

Amounts recommended are four or more servings each day from this vegetable-fruit group. These servings should include one good source of vitamin C (vitamin C is needed *daily*) or two servings of a fair source, and one serving, at least every other day, of a good source of vitamin A. The remaining servings may be any vegetable or fruit including those valuable in vitamins A and C.

Since orange juice is not allowed, finding a good source of vitamin C that your child likes sometimes is a problem. Fortified cranberry juice cocktail made into frozen popsicles is one solution. Children may not like just cranberry juice, but they do like the cranberry popsicles. As a last resort, it is possible to find vitamin C tablets that are uncolored and unflavored. Check with your doctor as to how much your child should take daily.

Milk Group

Foods included in the milk group are milk—whole, evaporated, skim, dry, and buttermilk—cheese—cottage, cream, Cheddar-type, or natural —ice cream, and yogurt.

Amounts recommended vary for different age groups. Children under nine should have two to three 8-ounce cups of whole milk; children nine to twelve should have three or more 8-ounce cups; and teenagers should have four or more 8-ounce cups. Part or all of the milk may be skim milk, buttermilk, evaporated milk, or dry milk. Other milk products may replace part of the milk as follows:

> 1-inch cube Cheddar-type cheese = ½ cup milk
> ½ cup yogurt = ½ cup milk
> ½ cup cottage cheese = ⅓ cup milk
> 2 tablespoons cream cheese = 1 tablespoon milk
> ½ cup ice cream or ice milk = ⅓ cup milk

Bread-Cereal Group

Foods included are all breads and cereals that are whole grained, enriched, or restored. This group includes, breads, cooked cereals, cold cereals, corn meal, crackers, flour, grits, macaroni, spaghetti, noodles, rice, rolled oats, and quick breads; and other baked goods if made with whole grain or enriched flour.

Amounts recommended are four servings or more daily. Count as one serving: one slice of bread, 1 ounce ready-to-eat cereal, ½ to ¾ cup cooked cereal, corn meal, grits, or pasta products.

APPENDIX E: Menus

Here are suggested menus for the first two weeks of the diet. We have kept the items rather general to allow flexibility. These menus strive for a well-balanced diet which must be kept in mind at all times.

Saturday 1
  Breakfast: Grapefruit juice
              Sausage patties (2x) (Make two times amount needed to provide some leftovers for future use.)
              Eggs
              Toast
              Milk
  Lunch: Hamburger on a bun
              Gelatin (2x)
              Potato Chips
              Milk
  Dinner: Chicken (3x) (save bones for soup)
              Potatoes (2x)
              Peas
              Carrot sticks
              Brownies (2x)
              Milk
  Snacks: Popsicles, cheese, peanuts, lemonade, or 7-Up

Sunday 1
  Breakfast: Waffles (2x and freeze)
              ½ grapefruit
              Carob milk
  Lunch: Chicken Soup
              Egg salad sandwich (hard boil extra eggs)
              Banana
              Milk
  Dinner: Roast beef or roast pork
              Asparagus or broccoli
              Potatoes

Rolls
Green salad
Pudding (2x)
Milk
Snacks: Cookies, celery with peanut butter, popcorn, pineapple
juice, or 7-Up

Monday 1
Breakfast: Pineapple juice
Eggs
Toast
Milk
Lunch: Chicken sandwich
Potato chips or peanuts
Gelatin salad or cottage cheese
Carob milk
Candy
Dinner: Meat loaf
Baked potato
Carrots
Slaw
Fruit in season or ice cream
Milk
Snacks: Fresh fruit, hard-boiled egg, peanut butter on crackers,
cranberry juice, or milk

Tuesday 1
Breakfast: Sausage patties
Eggs
½ grapefruit
Milk
Lunch: Roast beef or pork sandwich
Carrot sticks
Pudding
Cookies
Milk or small can of juice
Dinner: Chicken casserole
Squash or green beans
Cranberry gelatin
Rolls
Pie
Milk
Snacks: Cheese and crackers, fresh fruit, nuts, lemonade, or 7-
Up

Wednesday 1
  Breakfast: Banana
                 Eggs
                 Toast
                 Milk
  Lunch: Peanut butter and jelly sandwich
                 Brownies
                 Celery sticks
                 Milk shake
                 Candy
  Dinner: Fish
                 Potatoes
                 Broccoli or carrots
                 Green salad
                 Leftover pie with ice cream
                 Milk
  Snacks: Popsicles, Cracker Jack, cookies, grapefruit juice, or cranberry juice

Thursday 1
  Breakfast: Waffles
                 Grapefruit juice
                 Sausage patties
                 Milk
  Lunch: Leftover meat loaf sandwich
                 Cranberry gelatin
                 Carrot sticks
                 Brownies
                 Milk
  Dinner: Hamburger on a bun
                 French fries
                 Slaw
                 Cupcakes
                 Milk
  Snacks: Deviled egg, peanuts, fresh fruit, milk, or 7-Up

Friday 1
  Breakfast: ½ grapefruit or pineapple chunks
                 Eggs
                 Toast
                 Milk
  Lunch: Peanut butter and jelly or cheese sandwich
                 Carrot sticks or celery

	Banana
	Cupcake
	Milk
Dinner:	Pork or lamb chops
	Rice
	Pears or green beans
	Fruit salad
	Ice cream
Snacks:	Popcorn, cheese and crackers, cookies, lemonade, or 7-Up

Saturday 2

Breakfast:	Grapefruit juice
	Breakfast casserole (3x)
	Milk
Lunch:	Vegetable soup
	Tuna fish sandwich
	Pudding (2x)
	Milk
Dinner:	Chili (2x)
	Rolls
	Green salad
	Ice cream
	Milk
Snacks:	Cheese and crackers, cookies, fresh fruit, cranberry juice, or 7-Up

Sunday 2

Breakfast:	Banana
	French toast
	Sausage patties (2x)
	Milk
Lunch:	Egg salad sandwich
	Fruit gelatin
	Cupcake
	Milk shake
Dinner:	Roast beef
	Potatoes
	Corn
	Slaw salad
	Fruit cup
	Milk
Snacks:	Popcorn, lemonade, cookies, pineapple juice, or milk

Monday 2
  Breakfast: Pineapple chunks
               Eggs
               Toast
               Milk
  Lunch: Roast beef sandwich
               Banana
               Cookies
               Milk shake
  Dinner: Chicken (3x)
               Rice
               Peas
               Raw vegetable platter with dip
               Cupcakes (2x)
               Milk
  Snacks: Carrot sticks, cheese and crackers, pineapple juice,
               or ice cream

Tuesday 2
  Breakfast: ½ grapefruit
               Breakfast casserole
               Sweet rolls (2x)
               Milk
  Lunch: Chicken soup
               Peanut butter sandwich
               Potato chips
               Pudding
               Milk
  Dinner: Pork chops
               Potatoes
               Squash or spinach
               Slaw salad
               Pie
               Milk
  Snacks: Cupcakes, carrot sticks, fresh fruit, lemonade or milk
               shake

Wednesday 2
  Breakfast: Pineapple juice
               Eggs
               Sweet rolls
               Milk
  Lunch: Chicken sandwich
               Hard-boiled egg

Celery with peanut butter
Milk
Dinner: Fish
Potatoes
Carrots
Lettuce salad
Fruit in season or ice cream
Milk
Snacks: Cupcakes, cookies, peanuts, cranberry juice, or 7-Up

Thursday 2
Breakfast: Banana
Breakfast casserole
Milk
Lunch: Soup
Peanut butter and jelly sandwich
Potato chips
Carrot sticks
Pudding
Carob milk
Dinner: Chicken casserole
Broccoli
Slaw salad
Carob cake
Milk
Snacks: Cheese and crackers, celery stuffed with peanut butter,
Popsicles, 7-Up, or milk

Friday 2
Breakfast: Grapefruit juice
French toast
Sausage patties
Milk
Lunch: Chicken sandwich
Carrot sticks
Carob cake
Milk
Dinner: Hamburger on a bun
Baked beans
Lettuce salad
Fruit gelatin dessert
Milk
Snacks: Popcorn, fruit in season, potato chips, lemonade, or
7-Up

APPENDIX F: Equivalents

Here are some common conversions you may need:

Carob—Chocolate—Cocoa

   1 square of unsweetened chocolate = 3 tablespoons of carob powder

   1 tablespoon cocoa = 1 tablespoon carob powder

Unsalted Butter—Salted Butter

   Add about 1 teaspoon salt for each stick (½ cup) of uncolored
   butter used in a recipe

Fresh Onion—Dried Minced Onion

   1 tablespoon dried onion = ¼ cup raw onion

Dried Sweet Basil—Fresh Basil

   1 tablespoon dried crushed basil = about 6 to 8 tablespoons fresh
   chopped basil

Lemon Juice—Lemon Extract—Lemon Rind

   2 tablespoons fresh lemon juice = ½ teaspoon lemon extract = 1
   teaspoon grated rind

Index